The Pharmacopoeia of the United States of America

Facsimile of the first edition (1820)

American Institute of the History of Pharmacy
Madison, Wisconsin
2005

This facsimile of the first edition of the *Pharmacopoeia of the United States of America* (1820) is reproduced primarily from a copy held in the collections of the American Institute of the History of Pharmacy. A small number of pages are from a copy held by the Ebling Library of the University of Wisconsin, when necessary, due to damage, marginalia, or excess foxing. Every effort has been made to make the text reflect the original character of the first edition.

Production of this volume was supported through a grant received from the United States Pharmacopeial Convention, Inc. (USPC), Rockville, MD 20852.

Published by the American Institute of the History of Pharmacy, 777 Highland Ave., Madison, WI 53705

ISBN (cloth) 0-931292-40-9
ISBN (paper) 0-931292-41-7

THE

PHARMACOPŒIA

OF THE

UNITED STATES OF AMERICA.

1820.

BY THE
AUTHORITY OF THE MEDICAL SOCIETIES AND COLLEGES.

BOSTON:

PRINTED BY WELLS AND LILLY.
FOR CHARLES EWER, NO. 51, CORNHILL.
....
Dec. 1820.

In the General Medical Convention, held, in the Capitol at, Washington, January, 1820—

Resolved that

LYMAN SPALDING,
THOMAS T. HEWSON,
ELI IVES,
ELISHA DE BUTTS,
JACOB BIGELOW,

Be constituted a Committee whose duty it shall be to prepare for the Press the National Pharmacopœia agreed on in this Convention.

SAMUEL L. MITCHELL, *President.*

THOS. T. HEWSON, *Secretary.*

———

THE Pharmacopœia of the United States of America, is now published agreeably to the vote of the General Convention.

L. SPALDING,
Chairman of the Committee of Publication.

HISTORICAL INTRODUCTION.

As the authority and future usefulness of the American Pharmacopœia is connected with the manner in which this work has been formed; and as the extent of its adoption will probably be commensurate with that of the sources, from which it has emanated; it is proper to lay before the public an historical account of its origin, growth, and completion.

In January, 1817, Dr. Lyman Spalding submitted to the New York County Medical Society, a project for the formation of a National Pharmacopœia, by the authority of all the medical societies and medical schools in the United States. The plan proposed was, 1. That a convention should be called in each of the four grand divisions of the United States, to be composed of delegates from all the medical societies and schools. 2. That each district convention should form a Pharmacopœia, and elect delegates to meet in general convention in the city of Washington, on the first of January, 1820. 3. That the general convention should, from the district Pharmacopœias, form the national work. In the county medical society it was referred to a committee, who, after having corresponded with several of the leading medical men in each state, reported a set of resolutions, which were submitted to the medical society of the state of New York in February, 1818, and by them adopted and ordered to be carried into execution by a committee appointed for the purpose. The purport of these resolutions was as follows,

That it is expedient that a Pharmacopœia should be formed for the use of the United States.

That the several incorporated state medical societies, the several incorporated colleges of physicians and surgeons, or medical schools; and such medical bodies as constitute a faculty in any incorporated university or college in the United States, should be respectfully invited to unite in the formation of the American Pharmacopœia; and in case there should be any state or territory in the Union, in which there is no incorporated medical society, medical college, or school; that voluntary associations of physicians and surgeons, in such state or territory, be respectfully invited to unite in this undertaking.

That to form an American Pharmacopœia, it is expedient to divide the United States and territories into four districts, viz. the northern, middle, southern, and western.

That a convention be called in each of these districts.

That each state medical society, college of physicians and surgeons, medical school, faculty of medicine, and voluntary association, as before described, be invited to appoint one or more delegates to meet in a district convention.

That each district convention form a Pharmacopœia, or select one in general use, and make therein such alterations and additions as shall adapt it to the present state of medical science.

That each district convention be requested to appoint one or more delegates, to meet in a general convention, and submit to the same their Pharmacopœias.

That it be recommended to each medical society, &c. to defray the expenses of its own delegation, and its proportion of the expenses of the district convention.

That the general convention be held in the city of Washington on the first day of January, A. D. 1820, for the purpose of compiling the American Pharmacopœia from those Pharmacopœias which may be presented by the district conventions.

That the general convention adopt a plan for revising the American Pharmacopœia at the end of every ten years, and that no alteration be made therein except at those periods, and then only by the authority aforesaid.

That it be recommended to every medical society, &c. to adopt the American Pharmacopœia, and encourage the use of it by all druggists and apothecaries.

That the general convention sell, for ten years, the copy right of the American Pharmacopœia.

That the general convention defray their expenses out of the proceeds of the sale, and divide the surplus if any remain, equally among all the societies, &c. which were represented in the district conventions.

That this Society do now appoint David Hosack, M. D.; J. R. B. Rodgers, M. D.; Samuel L. Mitchell, M. D.; John Stearns, M. D.; John Watts, jun. M. D.; T. Romeyn Beck, M. D.; Lyman Spalding, M. D.; Wright Post, M. D.; and Alexander H. Stevens, M. D. delegates to meet in district convention, for the purpose of forming a Pharmacopœia.

That the delegates appointed by this Society be a special committee to correspond with all the incorporated state medical societies, &c. in the Union, and such influential medical men as they may deem proper.

That if a majority of the incorporated state medical societies, incorporated medical colleges, medical schools, and faculties of medicine, in the United States, approve of the formation of an American Pharmacopœia; that it be undertaken.

That when it shall be ascertained that a majority of the societies, &c. approve of the formation of a Pharmacopœia, the special committee of correspondence of the New York State Medical Society shall give public notice, as well as notice to all incorporated state medical societies, &c. that an American Pharmacopœia will be formed.

That in order to fix on times and places for holding the several district conventions, the special committee of correspondence be directed to request the several societies, &c. to name what time and place, in their opinion, would be most convenient for the meeting of the convention in their district; and when the formation of a Pharmacopœia is agreed on, that the aforesaid committee transmit to each society, &c. the names of the several places in their district, and the times which have been mentioned, and point out what time and place have the most votes, and submit to the several societies, &c. if such time and place would be most convenient.

That this society would propose the first day of June, A. D. 1819, and the city of Philadelphia, as a convenient time and place, for the meeting of the convention, in the district known by the name of the middle states.

The committee appointed by the New York medical society, on the 4th of March, 1818, issued circulars to the several corporate bodies and individuals designated in their commission. In reply to their first circular, information was received early in November, 1818, that the design of forming a National Pharmacopœia had met the approbation of a majority of the medical associations in the United States, and that they had appointed delegates to attend the district conventions. This intelligence was announced in a second circular, inviting the said associations to designate a time and place for the meeting of each of the district conventions: and in conformity therewith, the following places were designated, viz. Boston, Philadelphia, Columbia, S. C. and Lexington, Kentucky.

The VERMONT medical society at their annual meeting held in October, 1818, approved the formation of a National Pharmacopœia, and appointed Selah Gridley, M. D. and Erastus Torrey, M. D. their delegates.

The NEW HAMPSHIRE medical society approved the formation of a National Pharmacopœia on the 5th of May, 1819, and appointed the following delegates. Reuben D. Mussey, M. D.; Eben. Learned, M. D.; Matthias Spaulding, M. D.; and John P. Batchelder, M. D.

The MASSACHUSETTS medical society concurred in the formation of a National Pharmacopœia on the 2d day of June, 1818. They appointed John C. Warren, M. D.; John Gorham, M. D.; Jacob Bigelow, M. D.; James Thacher, M. D.; and George C. Shattuck, M. D. their delegates.

The RHODE ISLAND Medical society at their annual meeting held on the first of September, 1818, concurred in the formation of a National Pharmacopœia, and appointed Solomon Drowne, M. D. their delegate.

The medical faculty of BROWN University approved of the formation of a National Pharmacopœia on the 15th of March, 1819, and appointed William Ingalls, M. D. their delegate.

The CONNECTICUT medical society approved the design of forming a National Pharmacopœia, and on the 15th of October, 1818, appointed Eli Ives, M, D.; and William Tully, M. D. their delegates.

The faculty of the medical institution of YALE College on the 28th of October, 1818, approved the formation of an American Pharmacopœia, and appointed Nathan Smith, M. D.; and Eli Ives, M. D. their delegates.

The college of physicians and surgeons of the western district of the state of NEW YORK, in January, 1819, approved the formation of an American Pharmacopœia, and appointed Lyman Spalding, M. D. their delegate.

The college of physicians and surgeons in the city of NEW YORK on the 25th of June, 1818, approved the formation of the American Pharmacopœia, and appointed William James Mac Neven, M. D.; John W. Francis, M. D.; and Valentine Mott, M. D. their delegates.

The medical society of NEW JERSEY on the 11th of May, 1819, approved the formation of an American Pharmacopœia and appointed Charles Smith, M. D. and John Vancleve, M. D. their delegates.

The college of physicians of PHILADELPHIA, on the 2d day of February, 1819, approved the proposal for the formation of a National Pharmacopœia, and appointed Thomas Parke, M. D.; Samuel P. Griffiths, M. D.; Thomas C. James, M. D.; Thomas T. Hewson, M. D.; Edwin A. Atlee, M. D.; Samuel Stewart, M. D.; and Joseph Parrish, M. D. their delegates.

The medical society of the state of DELAWARE, in May, 1819, approved the formation of the national work, and appointed Joseph B. Harris, M. D., Allan M'Lane, jun. M. D., and William Baldwin, M. D. their delegates.

At the annual convention of the medical and chirurgical faculty of MARYLAND, in June, 1818. That body approved the formation of an American Phar-

macopœia, and appointed Nathaniel Potter, M. D.;
Elisha De Butts, M. D.; Samuel Baker, M. D.;
Henry Wilkins, M. D.; and Ennalls Martin, M. D.
their delegates.

The medical society of the district of COLUMBIA,
on the 5th of October, 1818, concurred in the plan
for a National Pharmacopœia, and appointed J. T.
Sheaffe, M. D. ; Thomas Sim, M. D.; Henry Huntt,
M. D.; and Thomas Henderson, M. D. their delegates.

The medical school at LEXINGTON, Ky. approved
the formation of a National Pharmacopœia, in April,
1819, and appointed B. W. Dudley, M. D.; and W.
H. Richardson, M. D. their delegates.

The medical college of OHIO approved the formation of the American Pharmacopœia, in July, 1819,
but on account of the infancy of their institution,
which had not then gone into complete operation,
they did not think proper to appoint delegates.

The board of physicians and surgeons of the first
medical district of the state of INDIANA on the 3d of
November, 1818, concurred in the formation of
an American Pharmacopœia, and appointed Elias
M'Narnee, M. D.; L. S. Shaler, M. D.; D. M.
Hale, M. D.; W. C. Whittesley, M. D.; and Philip
Barton, M. D. a committee to appoint delegates, &c.

The medical society of SOUTH CAROLINA, in Sep-
tember, 1818, approved the design of the American
Pharmacopœia, and appointed Joseph Johnson, M. D.;
John S. Trescott, M. D.; and James Moultrie, Jun.
M. D. their delegates.

The medical society of GEORGIA approved the formation of the National Pharmacopœia in May, 1819, and appointed Joel Abbot, M. D.; William Terrill, M. D.; J. B. Read, M. D.; and Jonas Cutter, M. D. their delegates.

The medical society of NEW ORLEANS approved in September, 1819, of the formation of the American Pharmacopœia, but their extreme distance from the place of meeting of either of the counties prevented them from sending delegates.

The delegates appointed to the district convention for the eastern states assembled in the Massachusetts Medical College at Boston, on the first day of June, 1819. At this meeting were present delegates from the medical societies of New Hampshire, Vermont, Massachusetts, Rhode Island, Connecticut, and from Brown University. The meeting was organized by the choice of John C. Warren, M. D. as chairman; and Jacob Bigelow, M. D. as secretary. A plan for a Pharmacopœia submitted by the delegates from Massachusetts, was taken up, and after being duly revised and amended, was adopted by this convention as their Pharmacopœia. Eli Ives, M. D.; and Jacob Bigelow, M. D. were appointed delegates to represent this convention in the general convention at Washington.

The district convention for the middle states met in the chamber of the College of Physicians in Philadelphia, on the first day of June, 1819. At this meeting were present delegates from the college of physicians of Philadelphia, the medical society of the

state of New York, the college of physicians and
surgeons of the city of New York; the college of
physicians and surgeons of the western district of New
York; the New Jersey medical society; the medical
and chirurgical faculty of Maryland; the medical
society of Delaware; and the medical society of the
District of Columbia. Thomas Parke, M. D. was
chosen president; Samuel L. Mitchell, M. D. vice
president; Lyman Spalding, M. D., and Samuel
Baker, M. D. secretaries. Two outlines of Pharmacopœias were submitted by the delegates from New
York and Philadelphia, out of which the committee
proceeded to form one, which was adopted as their
Pharmacopœia. The following gentlemen, viz. Samuel L. Mitchell, M. D.; Lyman Spalding, M. D.;
Alex. H. Stevens, M. D.; John Watts, M. D.;
Thomas T. Hewson, M. D., Thomas Parke, M. D.;
Allan M'Lane, M. D.; Elisha De Butts, M. D.;
Samuel Baker, M. D.; and Henry Huntt, M. D.
were appointed delegates to the General Convention
at Washington.

A quorum not being formed at the time and place
designated for the meeting of the southern district
convention, subsequent measures were taken by those
concerned, to secure effectually the representation of
that district in the General Convention at Washington.

The General Convention for the formation of the
American Pharmacopœia assembled in the Capitol at
Washington, on the first day of January, 1820, and
elected Samuel L. Mitchell, M. D. as their presi-

dent; and Thomas T. Hewson, M. D. as secretary. At this meeting, the northern, middle and southern districts were represented. Two Pharmacopœias, being those prepared in the northern and middle districts were submitted to examination by the respective delegates from those sections of the country. These works were duly examined and compared in detail, and their contents, with such additions as were thought necessary, consolidated into one work, which after full revision, was adopted by the General Convention as the American Pharmacopœia, and ordered to be published by a committee appointed for that purpose.

With a view to the future revision and republication of the Pharmacopœia, the following resolutions were adopted previously to the adjournment of the Convention.

Resolved, That in case of the death, resignation or inability to act, of the president of this Convention, that the secretary shall forthwith issue writs of election to the several delegates of this convention, who by written ballots addressed to him may elect another president.

Resolved, That in case of the death, &c. of the secretary, the president shall cause another to be elected as above described.

Resolved, That the president of this Convention shall, on the first of January, 1828, issue writs of election to the several incorporated state medical societies, &c. in the northern district, requiring them to ballot for three delegates to a General Convention to be held at Washington on the first of January, 1830, for the purpose of revising the American Pharmaco- pœia ; and that these several institutions be requested to forward to the president, on or before the first day of April, 1829, the names of three persons thus designated by ballot ; and the president of the Convention is here- by requested, on the said day, to assort and count the said votes, and to notify the three persons who shall have the greatest number of votes of their election ; and in case there should not be three persons who have a greater number of votes than others, then the said president is desired to put a ballot into the box for each of those persons who have an equal number of votes, and draw therefrom such number of ballots as shall make the number of delegates three, and notify as before.

This resolution to apply in like manner to the mid- dle, southern and western districts.

In case neither of the delegates from a district can attend, it shall be the duty of such delegates to ap- point a substitute who can attend.

Whereas the progressive improvements in medicine, as well as other causes, may render it expedient to revise the Pharmacopœia at an earlier period than is expressed above ; it shall be the duty of the president to call the attention of the medical societies and col- leges to the subject, whenever in his opinion the pub- lic good may require it.

PREFACE.

I⊤ is the object of a Pharmacopœia to select from among substances which possess medicinal power, those, the utility of which is most fully established and best understood ; and to form from them preparations and compositions, in which their powers may be exerted to the greatest advantage. It should likewise distinguish those articles by convenient and definite names, such as may prevent trouble or uncertainty in the intercourse of physicians and apothecaries.

The value of a Pharmacopœia depends upon the fidelity with which it conforms to the best state of medical knowledge of the day. Its usefulness depends upon the sanction it receives from the medical community and the public ; and the extent to which it governs the language and practice of those for whose use it is intended.

In most European countries works of this kind have appeared under the authority of medical colleges and corporations. Their usefulness has generally been co-extensive with the influence of the bodies of men from whom they have originated. If they have been less useful than might have been hoped from their

3

character and objects ; it is because different works of
this kind proceeding from different sources, and disa-
greeing with each other in their details, have been
permitted to circulate in the same community ; thus
interfering with each other, and frequently introduc-
ing confusion into the practice they were intended to
regulate.

In the United States the evil of irregularity and
uncertainty in the preparation of medicines has been
felt with peculiar weight. Besides a number of
Pharmacopœias, and of Dispensatories founded upon
them, which have been produced in different parts of
the Union ; we import various foreign works of the
kind, some of which have become naturalized by republication in the country. The druggist and the
medical practitioner are supplied, as their convenience
may direct, with any one or more of these books ; and
of course the character of medicinal preparations is lia-
ble to vary in every state and city of the Union. And
the physician is exposed, unconsciously, to administer
to his patient medicines, essentially different from
those which his judgment has prescribed.

That this evil has not earlier been remedied, is to
be attributed not so much to a want of conviction, on
the part of the medical faculty, of the importance of
the subject ; as to the difficulty of obtaining in such a
work the general co-operation of physicians throughout a country so extensive as ours. In several of the
states, measures had been taken by the faculty to regulate the preparation of medicines, and with success
as far as it respected the circle of their respective

practice.* But a National Pharmacopœia, which
should be established and adopted by the consent of
all the medical corporate bodies throughout the United States, still remained a great desideratum ; being
evidently the only mode by which a uniform system
could be introduced at once into all parts of the American territory. In the present volume a work of this
kind has for the first time been undertaken ; and after
being gradually matured by the advice, consent and
co-operation of bodies of physicians in all parts of the
Union, it is at length committed to the press, as the
result of their deliberations and decisions.

In the formation of the American Pharmacopœia,
the General Convention and their publishing committee have had to encounter those difficulties which
must always attend the first publication of works of
this kind. The selection of a Materia Medica ; the formation or adoption of preparations and compounds,
and the establishment of a pharmaceutical nomenclature, have constituted their chief labour. On each of
these departments of the work they have endeavoured to bestow that degree of careful inquiry and ma-
ture deliberation which the importance of the occasion demanded ; and have pursued the course, which
appeared to them best suited to supply the wants, and
promote the interests of the medical community in all
sections of the country.

* The Pharmacopœia of the Massachusetts Medical Society
was published in 1808, and afterwards adopted by the Medical
Society of New Hampshire. The Pharmacopœia of the New
York Hospital was published in 1816.

The fault of the lists of the Materia Medica which have been adopted in different countries, has always been their redundancy, rather than their deficiency. The number of articles necessary for the management of diseases, and especially of those which any individual physician actually employs; is always very far short of the catalogue afforded by most Pharmacopœias. Besides, as the progress of medical discovery continually tends to the introduction of new articles into use, the Materia Medica must soon grow to an unmanageable size, if its enlargement be not followed by a corresponding retrenchment of superfluities. In consequence of reasons of this sort, many articles contained in European books have been omitted in the American Pharmacopœia. These omissions have been made only where the articles in question were considered inert, or where they were abundantly superseded by substitutes more powerful and more accessible.

The system of retrenchment might no doubt have been more rigorously exercised without ultimate disadvantage to the interests of medicine. But it was thought to be at present more conducive to the public good, to retain on the list all those medicines which were believed to be so much in use in any part of the United States, that their omission would occasion inconvenience to physicians and apothecaries, and render the book less applicable to their wants.

In regard to indigenous vegetables, a considerable number, no doubt, possess important and useful properties; others have pretensions not yet fully settled.

But, as it happens in most countries, the number of simples occasionally employed in practice is much greater than it suits the proper compass of a Pharmacopœia to contain. In the present work, those native articles have been introduced which were considered to possess qualities sufficiently important, or which were found to be so much employed by practitioners, as to give them any claim to the character of standard medicines. In several instances native plants have been substituted for European ones of the same genus, where their qualities were esteemed the same.

With a view of discriminating between articles of decided reputation or general use, and those, the claims of which are of a more uncertain kind ; the Convention determined to refer to a secondary list such substances as were deemed of secondary or doubtful efficacy, retaining only on the principal list articles which might be considered of standard character. In the execution of this measure, particularly in the case of new medicines, they have possibly consigned to the secondary list some articles of more efficacy than others which they have retained on the primary one. In doubtful cases they have preferred to swell the subordinate rather than the primary catalogue, especially as this arrangement will be most likely to prompt farther investigations into the character of the substances in question.

In that part of the work which contains the formulæ for the preparations and compositions, the Convention have preserved those only which have received the sanction of the faculty in this country or in

Europe.   They have thought it their duty to insert
all which were reported to them by the District conventions, except in cases where the near similarity of
two preparations has rendered one of them super-
fluous.   Alterations of established formulæ have been
avoided, unless it be where the convenience and sim-
plicity of medicines could be promoted without
changing their operation or activity.

Those compound substances which are prepared
in the large way at manufactories, and which are to
be kept by the apothecary, though not necessarily
prepared by him, are inserted on the Materia Medica
list.   Those which are to be made by the apothecary
alone, are placed among the preparations and compositions.

It has been endeavoured that the *nomenclature*
adopted in this work should be conformable to the
present language of science, divested of as much of its
prolixity as can be done consistently with clearness
and distinctness.   It is conceded that the essential
properties of names ought to be expressiveness, brevity and dissimilarity.   Where these qualities can be
preserved without too great a departure from language
previously in use, they afford the best grounds of a
convenient and intelligible nomenclature.

In the designation of articles derived from the vegetable or animal kingdom, the Edinburgh college
has of late adopted the whole systematic name of the
plant or animal which affords the medicine.   The
London college has made use in most instances of a
shorter officinal name, in the genitive case, adding to

it the name of the part which is employed. In the American Pharmacopœia a single word is always used for the officinal name of the medicine wherever such a word is expressive, and without ambiguity. For example the name *Jalapa* is used instead of *Convolvulus Jalapa* of the Edinburgh Pharmacopœia, and *Jalapæ Radix* of the London ; *Colocynthis*, instead of *Cucumis Colocynthis* and *Colocynthidis Pulpa;* &c. The advantages of this mode are, that the name stands in the nominative case; that it expresses the medicine, and nothing else; that it is short and explicit, and does not require to be mutilated in practical use, as long names will inevitably be. The omission, in the Pharmaceutical name, of the word which expresses the part used, is not, as has been urged,* a sacrifice of propriety to brevity ; nor does it involve the alleged absurdity of transferring the name of the whole plant to one of its parts. The words *Jalapa*, *Ipecacuanha*, *Colocynthis*, *Senna*, and others of the same kind, are not, strictly speaking, the names of any plants, but the names of drugs and medicines. The substance which in English we call *Jalap*, is the root of a plant, the universally received scientific name of which is *Convolvulus Jalapa*. In strict accuracy, then, we must designate this drug by the circuitous name of *Convolvuli Jalapæ Radix*, or by the simple name of *Jalapa*.

* Translation of the London Pharmacopœia, 1815. Preface, page xii.

The chief advantage of the Edinburgh nomenclature is, that it points out accurately the source from which each substance is, or ought to be derived. The London college have in their last edition attained the same object by adding in a separate column the scientific term which indicates the source from which the medicine is procured. It has been thought best to pursue a similar plan in the American Pharmacopœia, and to dispose the Materia Medica in two columns, the first of which contains the officinal name in Latin and English ; while the second contains the corresponding scientific term, or the systematic name of the plant, animal or mineral, from which each substance is derived, with references for the sake of identification to authors who have described it ; a designation of the part to be used, and occasional explanations.

Brevity in the officinal names has been adhered to, wherever a distinct and expressive term was afforded by the common name of the article, or the generic or specific name of the plant or animal producing it. But in a few cases, single terms of this kind could not be employed without ambiguity, and it was thought better to adopt a double name previously in use, than to incur the evil of too great innovation by inventing a new word. This has happened where two parts of the same plant are used, as *Guaiaci lignum* and *Guaiaci resina ;* or where two plants occurred of the same genus, the specific names of which could not be used alone, as *Mentha piperita* and *Mentha viridis.* In some cases of this kind a single term has been applied by way of eminence to the article most used, and a

double name to one of inferior note, as *Gentiana* and
Gentiana Catesbœi.

The rule of brevity, and likewise the authority of
the latest Pharmacopœias, has in a small number of
individual cases been departed from, for sufficient reasons.   The motive has generally been a desire to preserve distinctness, and a preference to restore an old
name, rather than to adopt a new one which was
equivocal and partially received.

In the nomenclature of chemical substances the
Convention have followed the modern language of
chemistry, as it is most generally received at the present day.   They have pursued the example of the
London Pharmacopœia in placing the base of a compound body at the beginning of the name, this being
considered the most distinct way of presenting it.   A
few names of inconvenient length have been superseded by shorter terms, on previous pharmaceutical authority.   Under a like sanction, pharmaceutical names
have in a few instances been substituted for more accurate chemical ones, when the similarity of the latter
was considered to produce danger of mistake between
dissimilar substances.   This has been done particularly in the combinations of mercury with the muriatic
acid.

In the arrangement of the preparations and compositions, the alphabetical order of the subjects has been
adopted, as the most convenient method for reference.

Pharmacopœias have most frequently been published in the Latin language.   The Latin having long
been the common language of scientific men, and the

medium of technical phraseology, no well educated physician or apothecary is unacquainted with it. Its conciseness and precision have brought it into common use in the prescriptions of physicians and the formulæ of medical writers. From the weight due to considerations of this sort, the publishing committee, while they have written out the entire work in English, have thought it proper to present not only the nomenclature, but all the essential parts of the work in Latin also. They have further felt justified in this measure by the belief that the book is thus rendered more intelligible to foreigners, and more useful in those districts of the United States where the French and German languages continue to be spoken.

MATERIA MEDICA,

OR A CATALOGUE OF SIMPLE MEDICINES, TOGETHER WITH
SOME PREPARED MEDICINES, WHICH ARE KEPT IN THE
SHOP OF THE APOTHECARY, BUT NOT NECESSARILY PRE-
PARED BY HIM.

THE first column contains the officinal name of each article, in Latin and English. The second contains the corresponding scientific term, or the systematic name of the
animal or vegetable from which the medicine is derived;
likewise the part designated to be used, with the references
to authors and occasional explanations.

Abbreviations.—G. Gmelin, Edit. Systemæ Naturæ.—*W.* Willdenow, Edit. Spec.
Plantarum.—*L.* Linnæus.—*Mx.* Michaux Flora, Boreali-Americana.—*Muhl.*
Muhlenberg's Catalogue.—*Bw.* Bigelow's Medical Botany.—*Bn.* Barton's Vegetable Mat. Med.—*Oliv.* Olivier, Insectes Encycl. Methodique.—*Lond.* Pharmacopœia Londinensis, 1809.

ACACIÆ GUMMI.   Acacia vera. *W.* iv. 1085.
Acacia gum.   Mimosa Nilotica. *L.*
    Called *Gum Arabic.*   Gummi. *The Gum.*

ACETUM.   Acidum aceticum impurum.
Vinegar.

ACIDUM ARSENIOSUM.   Acidum arseniosum.
Arsenious acid.
    Called *White Arsenic.*

ACIDUM MURIATICUM. *Muriatic acid.*	**Acidum muriaticum.**
	The specific gravity to that of water as 1160 to 1000.
ACIDUM NITRICUM. *Nitric acid.*	**Acidum nitricum.**
	The specific gravity to that of water as 1500 to 1000.
ACIDUM SULPHURICUM. *Sulphuric acid.*	**Acidum sulphuricum.**
	The specific gravity to that of water as 1850 to 1000.
ACONITUM. *Aconite.*	**Aconitum neomontanum.** *W.* II. 1236. **Folia.** *The leaves.*
ADEPS. *Lard.*	**Sus scrofa.** G. 216. **Adeps.** *The lard.*
ALCOHOL. *Alcohol.*	**Alcohol.**
	The specific gravity to that of water as 835 to 1000.
ALLIUM. *Garlic.*	**Allium sativum.** *W.* II. 68. **Radix.** *The root.*
ALOE. *Aloes.*	
1. Aloe Socotrina. *Socotrine Aloes.*	Aloe spicata. *W.* II. 185. Extractum. *The extract.*
2. Aloe Barbadensis. *Barbadoes Aloes.*	Aloe vulgaris. *Lond.* 6. Extractum. *The extract.*

ALUMEN. *Alum.*	Super sulphas aluminæ et potassæ.
AMMONIACUM. *Ammoniacum.*	Heracleum gummiferum. *W. Hort.* *Berol.*——Gummi resina. *The* *Gum resin.*
AMMONIÆ MURIAS. *Muriate of ammonia.* Called *Sal Ammoniac.*	Ammoniæ murias.
AMYGDALA. *Almond.*	Amygdalus communis. *W.* II. 982. Nuclei. *The kernels.*
AMYGDALÆ OLEUM. *Oil of almonds.*	Amygdalus communis. Oleum fixum nucleorum. *The fix-* *ed oil of the kernels.*
ANGUSTURA. *Angustura.*	Bonplandia trifoliata. *W. Act. Be-* *rol.* 1802.—Cortex. *The bark.*
ANISUM. *Anise.*	Pimpinella anisum. *W.* I. 1473. Semina. *The seeds.*
ANTHEMIS. *Camomile.*	Anthemis nobilis. *W.* III. 2180. Flores. *The flowers.*
ANTIMONIUM. *Antimony.*	Antimonium.
ANTIMONII SULPHURETUM. *Sulphuret of antimony.*	Antimonii sulphuretum.
AQUA. *Water.*	Aqua fontana.

ARGENTUM.
Silver.

Argentum.

ARMORACIA.
Horse radish.

Cochlearia armoracia. *W.* III. 451.
Planta. *The plant.*

ASSAFŒTIDA.
Assafetida.

Ferula Assafœtida. *W.* I. 1413.
Gummi resina. *The gum resin.*

AURANTII CORTEX.
Orange peel.

Citrus aurantium. *W.* III. 1427.
Cortex fructûs. *The rind of the
    fruit.*

AURUM.
Gold.

Aurum.

AVENÆ FARINA.
Oatmeal.

Avena sativa. *W.* I. 446.
Farina. *The meal.*

BARYTÆ SULPHAS.
Sulphate of baryta.

Barytæ sulphas.

BELLADONNA.
Deadly nightshade.

Atropa belladonna. *W.* I. 1017.
Folia. *The leaves.*

BENZOINUM.
Benzoin.

Styrax benzoin. *W.* II. 623.
Balsamum. *The balsam.*

BISMUTHUM.
Bismuth.

Bismuthum.

CAJUPUTI OLEUM.
Cajuput oil.

Melaleuca cajuputi. *Lond.* 8.
Oleum volatile. *The volatile oil.*

CALX.
Lime.

Calx.

CALCIS CARBONAS. Calcis carbonas.
Carbonate of lime.
 1. Durus, *Hard*, called *Marble.*
 2. Mollis, *Soft*, called *Chalk.*

CALCIS PHOSPHAS. Calcis phosphas.
Phosphate of lime.

CAMPHORA. Laurus camphora. W. II. 478. *also*
Camphor. Dryobalanops camphora *Cole-*
  brooke, Asiatic Researches, XII.
  535.—Camphora. *The camphor.*

CANELLA. Canella alba. *W.* II. 851.
Canella. Cortex. *The bark.*

CANTHARIDES. Cantharis vesicatorius. *Oliv.*V. 277.
Cantharides. Meloe vesicatorius. *L.*
 Lytta vesicatoria. *Fabricius.*

CANTHARIDES VITTATÆ. Cantharis vittata. *Oliv.* V. 279.
Potato flies. Lytta vittata. *Fabricius.*

CAPSICUM. Capsicum annuum. *W.* I. 1050.
Cayenne pepper. Fructus. *The fruit.*

CARBO LIGNI. Carbo ligni.
Charcoal.

CARDAMOMUM. Amomum repens. *W.* I. 9.
Cardamom. Elettaria cardamomum. *Maton Tr.*
  Lin. Soc.—Semina. *The seeds.*

CARUM. Carum carui. *W.* I. 1470.
Caraway. Semina. *The seeds.*

CARYOPHYLLI. Eugenia caryophyllata. *W.* III. 965.
Cloves. Gemmæ florales. *The flower buds.*

CARYOPHYLLORUM OLEUM. Eugenia caryophyllata.
Oil of cloves. Oleum volatile. *The volatile oil.*

CASCARILLA. Croton Eleutheria. *W.* IV. 546.
Cascarilla. Cortex. *The bark.*

CASSIA FISTULA. Cassia fistula. *W.* II. 518.
Purging cassia. Pulpa. *The pulp of the pods.*

CASSSA MARILANDICA. Cassia marilandica. *W.* II. 524.
American senna. *Bw.* II. 166. *Bn.* I. 137.
  Planta. *The plant.*

CASTOREUM. Castor fiber. *G.* 124.
Castor. Castoreum. *The castor.*

CATECHU. Acacia catechu. *W.* IV. 1079.
Catechu. Mimosa catechu. *L.*
  Extractum. *The extract.*

CERA. Apis mellifica.
Wax. Favus fusus. *The melted comb.*
  1. Flava. *Yellow.*
  2. Alba. *White.*

CEREVISIÆ FERMENTUM. Cerevisiæ fermentum.
Yeast.

CHENOPODIUM. Chenopodium anthelminticum. *W.*
Wormseed. I. 1304. *Bn.* II. 183.
  Planta. *The plant.*

CINCHONA.
Peruvian bark.

1. Cinchona pallida.	Cinchona lancifolia. *Lond.* 10.
Pale bark.	Cortex. *The bark.*
2. Cinchona rubra.	Cinchona oblongifolia. *Lond.* 10.
Red bark.	Cortex. *The bark.*
3. Cinchona flava.	Cinchona cordifolia. *Lond.* 10.
Yellow bark.	Cortex. *The bark.*

CINNAMOMUM.   Laurus cinnamomum. *W.* II. 477.
Cinnamon.   Cortex. *The bark.*

CINNAMOMI OLEUM.   Laurus cinnamomum.
Oil of cinnamon.   Oleum volatile. *The volatile oil.*

COLCHICUM.   Colchicum autumnale. *W.* II. 272.
Meadow saffron.   Radix. *The root.*

COLOCYNTHIS.   Cucumis colocynthis. *W.* IV. 611.
Colocynth.   Fructus, cortice seminibusque abjectis. *The fruit deprived of its rind and seeds.*

COLOMBA.
Columbo.   Radix. *A root. The plant unknown.*

CONIUM.   Conium maculatum. *W.* I. 1395.
Hemlock.   *Bw.* I. 113.
Folia. *The leaves.*

COPAIBA.   Copiafera officinalis. *W.* II. 630.
Copaiba.   Balsamum. *The balsam.*

5

CORIANDRUM.	Coriandrum sativum. *W.* I. 1443.
Coriander.	Semina. *The seeds.*

CORNU CERVI.	Cervus elaphus. *G.* 176.
Stag's horn.	Cornua. *The horns.*

CORNUS FLORIDA.	Cornus florida. *W.* I. 661. *Bw.*
Dogwood.	II. 73. *Bn.* I. 44.
	Cortex. *The bark.*

CROCUS.	Crocus sativus. *W.* I. 194.
Saffron.	Stigmata. *The stigmas.*

CUBEBA.	Piper cubeba. *W.* I. 159.
Cubebs.	Fructus. *The fruit.*

CUPRUM.	Cuprum.
Copper.	

CUPRI SUBACETAS.	Cupri subacetas.
Subacetate of copper.	
Called *Verdigris.*	

CUPRI SULPHAS.	Cupri sulphas.
Sulphate of copper.	
Called *Blue Vitriol.*	

DIGITALIS.	Digitalis purpurea. *W.* III. 283.
Foxglove.	Folia. *The leaves.*

DOLICHOS.	Dolichos pruriens. *W.* III. 283.
Cowhage.	Pubes leguminis. *The bristles of*
	the pod.

DRACONTIUM.   Dracontium fœtidum. *W.* II. 288.
Skunk cabbage.   Ictodes fœtidus. *Bw.* II. 41.
    Symplocarpus fœtidus. *Bn.* I. 123.
    Radix. *The root.*

DULCAMARA.   Solanum dulcamara. *W.* I. 1028.
Bitter sweet.   *Bw.* I. 169.
    Stipites. *The stalks.*

ELATERIUM.   Momordica elaterium. *W.* IV. 605.
Elaterium.   Extractum fructus. *The extract of*
    the fruit. Lond.

EUPATORIUM PERFOLIA- Eupatorium perfoliatum. *W.* III.
TUM.   1761. *Bw.* I. 38. *Bn.* II. 125.
Thoroughwort.   Herba. *The herb.*

EUPATORIUM TEUCRIFO- Eupatorium teucrifolium. *W.* III.
LIUM.   1753.
Wild horehound.   Herba. *The herb.*

EUPHORBIA IPECACUAN- Euphorbia ipecacuanha. *W.* II.
HA.   900. *Bw.* III. 109. *Bn.* I. 211.
Ipecacuanha spurge.   Radix. *The root.*

EUPHORBIA COROLLATA. Euphorbia corollata. *W.* II. 916.
Large flowering spurge.   *Bw.* III. 118.
    Radix. *The root.*

FERRUM.   Ferrum.
Iron.

FERRI PRUSSIAS.   Ferri prussias.
Prussiate of iron.

FERRI SULPHAS.
Sulphate of iron.

Ferri sulphas.

FICUS.
Figs.

Ficus carica. *W.* IV.
Fructus. *The fruit.*

FŒNICULUM.
Fennel.

Anethum fœniculum. *W.* I. 1469.
Semina. *The seeds.*

FRASERA.
American columbo.

Frasera Walteri. *Mx.* I. 96. *Bn.*
II. 103.
Radix. *The root.*

GALBANUM.
Galbanum.

Bubon galbanum. *W.* I. 1439.
Gummi resina. *The gum resin.*

GALLÆ.
Galls.

Quercus cerris. *W.* IV. 454.
Cyniphis nidus. *The nest of Cynips*
Quercifolii.

GAMBOGIA.
Gamboge.

Stalagmitis cambogioides.
Gummi resina. *The gum resin.*
Obtained also from some other
vegetables.

GENTIANA.
Gentian.

Gentiana lutea. *W.* I. 1331.
Radix. *The root.*

GERANIUM.
Cranesbill.

Geranium maculatum. *W.* III. 705.
Bw. I. 84. *Bn.* I. 149.
Radix. *The root.*

GILLENIA. | Gillenia trifoliata. *Bw.* III. 10.
Gillenia. | *Bn.* I. 65.
Spiræa trifoliata. *W.* II. 1063.
Radix. *The root.*

GLYCYRRHIZÆ RADIX. | Glycyrrhiza glabra. *W.* III. 1144.
Liquorice root. | Radix. *The root.*

GLYCYRRHIZÆ EXTRAC-Glycyrrhiza glabra.
TUM. | Extractum. *The extract.*
Extract of liquorice.

GUAIACI LIGNUM. | Guaiacum officinale. *W.* II. 508.
Guaiacum wood. | Lignum. *The wood.*
Called *Lignum vitæ.*

GUAIACI RESINA. | Guiacum officinale.
Resin of guaiacum. | Resina. *The resin.*

HÆMATOXYLON. | Hæmatoxylon campechianum. *W.*
Logwood. | II. 547.
Lignum. *The wood.*

HELLEBORUS FŒTIDUS. | Helleborus fœtidus. *W.* II. 1337.
Bearsfoot. | Folia. *The leaves.*

HELLEBORUS NIGER. | Helleborus niger. *W.* II. 1336.
Black hellebore. | Radix. *The root.*

HEUCHERA. | Heuchera cortusa. *Mx.* I. 171.
Alum root. | *Bn.* II. 159.
Heuchera Americana. *W.* I. 1328.
Radix. *The root.*

HORDEUM.　　Hordeum distichon.　*W.* I. 473.
Barley.　　Semina decorticata.　*The seeds de-*
　　　　　　　　corticated.

HUMULUS.　　Humulus lupulus.　*W.* IV. 769.
Hop.　　　　*Bw.* III. 162.
　　　　　　Strobili.　*The strobiles.*

HYDRARGYRUM.　　Hydrargyrum.
Mercury.

HYOSCYAMUS.　　Hyoscyamus niger.　*W.* I. 1010.
Henbane.　　　*Bw.* II. 161.
　　　　　　　Planta.　*The plant.*

ICTHYOCOLLA.　　Accipenser huso, *and some other*
Isinglass.　　　*species.*—Vesica natoria.　*The*
　　　　　　　　swimming bladder.

INULA.　　Inula helenium.　*W.* III. 2089.
Elecampane.　　Radix.　*The root.*

IPECACUANHA.　　Callicocca ipecacuanha.　*Brotero.*
Ipecacuanha.　　*Lin. Trans.* VI.　137.
　　　　　　　Radix.　*The root.*

JALAPA.　　Convolvulus jalapa.　*W.* I. 860.
Jalap.　　Radix.　*The root.*

JUGLANS.　　Juglans cinerea.　*W.* IV.　456.
Butternut.　　*Bw.* II. 115.
　　　　　　Liber radicis.　*The inner bark of*
　　　　　　the root.

JUNIPERUS.   Juniperus communis.   *W.* IV. 855.
Juniper.   *Bw.* III. 45.
             Baccæ.   *The berries.*

JUNIPERUS VIRGINIANA.   Juniperus virginiana.   *W.* IV. 863.
Red cedar.   *Bw.* III. 50.
             Folia.   *The leaves.*

KINO.   Pterocarpus.——*Mungo Park : last*
Kino.   *Journal,* p. cxxiv.
             E·..actum.   *The extract.*   *Also*
             from other plants.

LACTUCARIUM.   Lactuca sativa.   *W.* III. 1523.
Lactucarium.   Succus concretus.   *The concrete*
             juice.

LAURUS CASSIA.   Laurus ,cassia.   *W.* II. 477.
Cassia bark.   Cortex.   *The bark.*

LAVANDULA.   Lavandula spica.   *W.* III. 60.
Lavender.   Flores.   *The flowers.*

LICHEN.   Lichen Islandicus.
Iceland moss.   Planta.   *The plant.*

LIMON.   Citrus medica.   *W.* III. 1426.
Lemon.   Fructus.   *The fruit.*

LIMONIS OLEUM.   Citrus medica.
Oil of lemon.   Oleum volatile corticis fructus.   *The*
             volatile oil of the rind of the fruit.

LINI SEMINA.   Linum usitatissimum.   *W.* I. 1533.
Flaxseed.   Semina.   *The seeds.*

LINI OLEUM. *Flaxseed oil.* Called *Linseed Oil.*	Linum usitatissimum. Oleum fixum seminis. *The fixed oil of the seeds.*
LIRIODENDRON. *Tulip tree.*	Liriodendron tulipifera. *W.* II. 1254. *Bw.* II. 107. *Bn.* I. 92. Cortex. *The bark.*
LOBELIA. *Indian tobacco.*	Lobelia inflata. *W.* I. 046. *Bw.* 177. *Bn.* I. 181. Herba. *The herb.*
MAGNESIÆ CARBONAS. *Carbonate of magnesia.*	Magnesiæ carbonas.
MAGNESIÆ SULPHAS. *Sulphate of magnesia.* Called *Epsom Salt.*	Magnesiæ sulphas.
MANNA. *Manna.*	Fraxinus ornus. *W.* IV. 1104. Succus concretus. *The concrete juice.*
MARANTA. *Arrow root.*	Maranta arundinacea. *W.* I. 13. Fœcula radicis. *The fecula of the root.*
MEL. *Honey.*	Apis mellifica. Mel. *The honey.*
MENTHA PIPERITA. *Peppermint.*	Mentha piperita. *W.* III. 79. Herba. *The herb.*
MENTHA VIRIDIS. *Spear mint.*	Mentha viridis. *W.* III. 76. Herba. *The herb.*

MEZEREON.
Mezereon.

Daphne mezereon. *W.* II. 415.
Cortex radicis. *The bark of the root.*

MOSCHUS.
Musk.

Moschus moschiferus. *G.* 172.
Moschus. *The musk.*

MYRISTICA.
Nutmeg.

Myristica moschata. *W.* IV. 869.
Nucleus. *The kernel of the fruit.*

MYRISTICÆ OLEUM.
Oil of nutmeg.
Called *Oil of mace.*

Myristica moschata.
Oleum nuclei fixo-volatile. *The compound oil of the kernel.*

MYROXYLON.
Balsam of Peru.

Myroxylon Peruiferum. *W.* II. 546.
Balsamum. *The balsam.*

MYRRHA.
Myrrh.

Gummi-resina. *A gum resin. The tree unknown.*

NUX VOMICA.
Vomic nut.

Strychnos nux vomica. *W.* I. 1052.
Semina. *The seeds.*

OLIVÆ OLEUM.
Olive oil.

Olea Europæa. *W.* I. 44.
Oleum fructus. *The oil of the fruit.*

OPIUM.
Opium.

Papaver somniferum. *W.* II. 1147.
Succus concretus. *The concrete juice.*

ORIGANUM.
Wild marjoram.

Origanum vulgare. *W.* III. 135.
Herba. *The herb.*

6

PHOSPHORUS. *Phosphorus.*	Phosphorus.
PHYTOLACCA. *Poke.*	Phytolacca decandra. *W.* II. 822. *Bw.* I. 39. *Bn.* II. 213. Radix. *The root.*
PIMENTA. *Pimento.*	Myrtus Pimenta. *W.* II. 973. Baccæ. *The berries.*
PIPER. *Black pepper.*	Piper nigrum. *W.* I. 159. Baccæ. *The berries.*
PIX ABIETIS. *Burgundy pitch.*	Pinus abies. *W.* IV. 506. Resina præparata. *The prepared resin.*
PIX LIQUIDA. *Tar.*	Pinus palustris. *W.* IV. 499. *and some other species.*—Terebin- thina empyreumatica. *The im- pure turpentine procured by burn- ing.*
PLUMBUM. *Lead.*	Plumbum.
PLUMBI OXYDUM SEMIVI- TREUM. *Semivitrified oxide of lead.* Called *Litharge.*	Plumbi oxidum semivitreum.
PLUMBI SUBCARBONAS. *Subcarbonate of lead.* Called *White lead.*	Plumbi subcarbonas.

PODOPHYLLUM.
May apple.

Podophyllum peltatum. *W.* II.
1141. *Bw.* II. 34. *Bn.* II. 9.
Radix. *The root.*

POTASSÆ NITRAS.
Nitrate of potass.
Called *Nitre.*

Potassæ nitras.

POTASSÆ SUBCARBONAS
IMPURUS.
*Impure subcarbonate of
potass.*
Called *Pearl ask.*

Potassæ subcarbonas impurus.

POTASSÆ SUPERTARTRAS.
Supertartrate of potass.
Called *Cream of Tartar.*

Potassæ supertartras.

PRUNA.
Prunes.

Prunus domestica. *W.* II. 896.
Fructus siccatus. *The dried fruit.*

PYRETHRUM.
Pellitory of Spain.

Anthemis Pyrethrum. *W.* III. 2184.
Radix. *The root.*

QUASSIA.
Quassia.

Quassia excelsa. *W.* II. 569.
Lignum. *The wood.*

QUERCUS ALBA.
White oak.

Quercus alba. *W.* IV. 448.
Cortex. *The bark.*

QUERCUS TINCTORIA.
Black oak.

Quercus tinctoria. *W.* IV. 444.
Cortex. *The bark.*

RESINA PINI. *Pine resin.*	Pinus palustris,&c. *W.* IV. 499,&c. Terebinthina oleo dempto. *The* *residuum after the distillation of* *oil of turpentine.*
RHAMNUS. *Buckthorn.*	Rhamnus catharticus. *W.* I. 1092, Baccæ. *The berries.*
RHEUM. *Rhubarb.*	Rheum palmatum. *W.* II. 489. Radix. *The root.*
RICINI OLEUM. *Castor oil.*	Ricinus communis. *W.* IV. 564. Oleum fixum seminis. *The fixed* *oil of the seed.*
ROSA. *Rose.*	Rosa centifolia. *W.* II. 1071. Petala. *The petals.*
ROSMARINUS. *Rosemary.*	Rosmarinus officinalis. *W.* I. 126. Cacumina. *The tops.*
SABBATIA. *American centaury.*	Sabbatia angularis. *Bw.* III. 56. *Bn.* I. 255.—Chironia angularis. *L.*—Planta. *The plant.*
SABINA. *Savin.*	Juniperus sabina. *W.* IV. 852. Folia. *The leaves.*
SACCHARUM. *Sugar.*	Saccharum officinarum. *W.* I. 321. Saccharum purificatum. *The re-* *fined sugar.*
SAGO. *Sago.*	Cycas circinalis. Medulla. *The pith.*

SALEP. *Salep.*	Orchis mascula. *W.* IV. 18. and Orchis morio.—Fœcula radicis. *The fecula of the root.*
SALIX. *Willow.*	Salix eriocephala. *Mx.* II. 225. *and* *some other species.* Cortex. *The bark.*
SAMBUCUS. *Elder.*	Sambucus Canadensis. *W.* I. 1494. Baccæ. *The berries.*
SANGUINARIA. *Bloodroot.*	Sanguinaria Canadensis. *W.* II. 1140. *Bw.* I. 75. *Bn.* I. 31. Radix. *The root.*
SAPO. *Castile soap.*	Sapo Hispanicus.
SARSAPARILLA. *Sarsaparilla.*	Smilax sarsaparilla. *W.* IV. 776. Radix. *The root.*
SASSAFRAS. *Sassafras.*	Laurus sassafras. *W.* II. 485. *Bw.* II. 142. Cortex radicis. *The bark of the root.*
SCAMMONIUM. *Scammony.*	Convolvulus scammonia. *W.* I. 845. Gummi resina. *The gum resin.*
SCILLA. *Squill.*	Scilla maritima. *W.* II. 125. Radix. *The root.*
SENEGA. *Seneca snake root.*	Polygala senega. *W.* III. 894. *Bw.* II. 97. *Bn.* II. 111. Radix. *The root.*

SENNA.   Cassia senna. *W.* II. 520.
Senna.   Folia. *The leaves.*

SERPENTARIA.   Aristolochia Serpentaria. *W.* IV.
Virginia snake root.   159. *Bw.* III. 62. *Bn.* II. 41.
                        Radix. *The root.*

SEVUM.   Ovis aries. *G.* 197.
Suet.   Sevum. *The suet.*

SIMAROUBA.   Quassia simarouba. *W.* II. 568.
Simarouba.   Cortex. *The bark.*

SINAPIS.   Sinapis nigra. *W.* III. 555.
Mustard.   Semina. *The seeds.*

SODÆ MURIAS.   Sodæ murias.
Muriate of soda.
    Called *Sea salt.*

SODÆ SUBBORAS.   Sodæ subboras.
Subborate of soda.
    Called *Borax.*

SODÆ SUBCARBONAS.   Sodæ subcarbonas.
Subcarbonate of soda.

SODÆ SULPHAS.   Sodæ sulphas.
Sulphate of soda.
    Called *Glaubers salt.*

SPERMACETI.   Physeter macrocephalus. *G.* 227.
Spermaceti.   Spermaceti. *The spermaceti.*

SPIGELIA.
Carolina pink.

Spigelia marilandica. *W.* I. 825.
Bw. I. 142. *Bn.* II. 75.
Planta. *The plant.*

SPONGIA.
Sponge.

Spongia officinalis. *G.* 3820.

STANNUM.
Tin.

Stannum.

STATICE.
Marsh rosemary.

Statice Caroliniana. *Walter Flor.*
Car. 118. *Bw.* II. 51.
Radix. *The root.*

STRAMONIUM.
Thorn apple.

Datura stramonium. *W.* I. 1008.
Bw. I. 17.
Folia. *The leaves.*

STRAMONII SEMINA.
Thorn apple seeds.

Datura stramonium.
Semina. *The seeds.*

SUCCINUM.
Amber.

Succinum.

SULPHUR.
Sulphur.

Sulphur sublimatum et lotum.

TABACUM.
Tobacco.

Nicotiana tabacum. *W.* I. 1014.
Bw. II. 171.
Folia. *The leaves.*

TAMARINDUS.
Tamarind.

Tamarindus Indica. *W.* III. 577.
Fructus conditus. *The preserved fruit.*

TAPIOCA. *Tapioca.*	Jatropha manihot. *W.* IV. 562. Fœcula radicis. *The fecula of the root.*
TEREBINTHINA. *Turpentine.*	Pinus palustris, &c. *W.* IV. 499. &c. Terebinthina. *The turpentine.*
TEREBINTHINÆ OLEUM. *Oil of turpentine.*	Ejusdem oleum volatile. *The volatile oil of the preceding article.*
TEREBINTHINA CANADENSIS. *Canada balsam.*	Pinus balsamea. *W.* IV. 504. Balsamum. *The balsam.*
TOLUTANUM. *Tolu.*	Toluifera balsamum. *W.* II. 545. Balsamum. *The balsam.*
TRAGACANTHA. *Tragacanth.*	Astragalus verus. *Lond.* 49. Gummi. *The gum.*
ULMUS. *Slippery elm.*	Ulmus fulva. *Mx.* I. 172. Liber. *The inner bark.*
UVÆ. *Raisins.*	Vitis vinifera. *W.* I. 1180. Fructus siccatus. *The dried fruit.*
UVA URSI. *Uva ursi.*	Arbutus uva ursi. *W.* II. 618. *Bw.* I. 66. Folia. *The leaves.*
VALERIANA. *Valerian.*	Valeriana officinalis. *W.* I. 177. Radix. *The root.*

VERATRUM ALBUM.
White hellebore.

Veratrum album. *W.* IV. 895.
Radix. *The root.*

VERATRUM VIRIDE.
American hellebore.

Veratrum viride. *W.* IV. 896.
Bw. II. 121.
Radix. *The root.*

VINUM.
Wine.

Vitis vinifera. *W.* I. 1180.
Vinum. *The wine. The sort called Teneriffe.*

WINTERA.
Winter's bark.

Wintera aromatica. *W.* II. 1239.
Cortex. *The bark.*

XANTHORHIZA.
Yellow root.

Xanthorhiza apiifolia. *W.* I. 1568.
Bn. II. 203.
Radix. *The root.*

XANTHOXYLUM.
Prickly ash.

Xanthoxylum fraxineum. *W.* IV.
754. *Bw.* III. 156.
Cortex. *The bark.*

ZINCUM.
Zinc.

Zincum.

ZINCI CARBONAS IMPURUS. Zinci carbonas impurus.
Impure carbonate of zinc.
Called *Calamine.*

ZINCI OXIDUM IMPURUM. Zinci oxidum impurum.
Impure oxide of zinc.
Called *Tutty.*

7

ZINCI SULPHAS.   Zinci sulphas.
Sulphate of zinc.
    Called *White vitriol.*

ZINGIBER.   Amomum zingiber.   *W.* I. 6.
Ginger.   Zingiber officinale.   *Roscoe Lin.*
         Trans.—Radix.   *The root.*

SECONDARY LIST.

ALETRIS.
Star grass.

Aletris farinosa. *W.* II. 183. *Bw.*
III. 94.
Radix. *The root.*

ANGELICA.
Angelica.

Angelica atropurpurea. *W.* I. 1430.
Planta. *The plant.*

APOCYNUM.
Dog's bane.

Apocynum androsæmifolium. *W.*
I. 1259. *Bw.* II. 148.
Radix. *The root.*

ARALIA NUDICAULIS.
False sarsaparilla.

Aralia nudicaulis. *W.* I. 1521.
Radix. *The root.*

ARALIA SPINOSA.
Angelica tree.

Aralia spinosa. *W.* I. 1521.
Cortex. *The bark.*

ARNICA.
Leopard's bane.

Arnica montana. *W.* III. 2106.
Planta. *The plant.*

ARUM.
Dragon root.

Arum triphyllum. *W.* IV. 480.
Bw. I. 52.
Radix. *The root.*

ASARUM.   Asarum Canadense. *W.* II. 838.
Canada snake root.   *Bw.* I. 49. *Bn.* II. 85.
                     Radix. *The root.*

ASCLEPIAS INCARNATA. Asclepias incarnata. *W.* I. 1267.
Flesh coloured asclepias. Radix. *The root.*

ASCLEPIAS SYRIACA.   Asclepias Syriaca. *W.* I. 1265.
Common silk weed.   Radix. *The root.*

ASCLEPIAS TUBEROSA. Asclepias tuberosa. *W.* I. 1268.
Butterfly weed.   *Bw.* II. 59. *Bn.* I. 239.
                     Radix. *The root.*

AZEDARACH.   Melia azedarach. *W.* II. 558.
Azedarach.   Cortex. *The bark.*

BITUMEN.   Bitumen.
Bitumen.

CALAMUS.   Acorus calamus. *W.* II. 199.
Sweet flag root.   *Bn.* II. 63.
                     Radix. *The root.*

CAROTA.   Daucus carota. *W.* I. 1389.
Carrot.   Semina. *The seed.*

CARTHAMUS.   Carthamus tinctorius. *W.* III. 1706.
Dyer's saffron.   Flores. *The flowers.*

CASTANEA.   Castanea pumila. *W.* IV. 461.
Chinquapin.   Cortex. *The bark.*

CIMICIFUGA.
Black snake root.

Cimicifuga serpentaria. *Pursh.* II.
382.—Radix. *The root.*

CONTRAYERVA.
Contrayerva.

Dorstenia contrayerva. *W.* I. 688.
Radix. *The root.*

CONVOLVULUS PANDURA-
TUS.
Wild potatoe.

Convolvulus panduratus. *W.* I.
850. *Bn.* I. 249.
Radix. *The root.*

CORNUS CIRCINATA.
Round leaved dogwood.

Cornus circinata. *W.* I. 663.
Cortex. *The bark.*

CORNUS SERICEA.
Swamp dogwood.

Cornus sericea. *W.* I. 663. *Bn.*
I. 115.—Cortex. *The bark.*

COPTIS.
Goldthread.

Coptis trifolia. *Salisbury. Lin.*
Tr. VIII. 305. *Bw.* I. 60. *Bn.*
II. 97.—Radix. *The root.*

COTULA.
May weed.

Anthemis cotula. *W.* III. 2181.
Bn. I. 161.
Planta. *The plant.*

CURCUMA.
Turmeric.

Curcuma longa. *W.* I. 14.
Radix. *The root.*

DELPHINIUM.
Larkspur.

Delphinium consolida. *W.* II. 1226.
Radix. *The root.*

DIOSPYROS.
Persimmon.

Diospyros Virginiana. *W.* IV. 1107.
Cortex. *The bark.*

ERIGERON CANADENSE.
Canada flea bane.

Erigeron Canadense. *W.* III. 1954.
Planta. *The plant.*

ERIGERON PHILADELPHI-　Erigeron Philadelphicum.　*W.* III.
　　CUM.　　　　　　　　1957.　*Bn.* I. 227.
Philadelphia flea bane.　Planta.　*The plant.*

ERYNGIUM.　　　　　　Eryngium aquaticum.　*W.* I. 1357.
Button snake root.　　Radix.　*The root.*

ERYTHRONIUM.　　　　Erythronium Americanum.　*Muhl.*
Erythronium.　　　　　84.　*Bw.* III. 151.
　　　　　　　　　　　Planta.　*The plant.*

EUPATORIUM PURPUREUM.　Eupatorium purpureum.　*W.* III.
Gravel root.　　　　　1759.—Radix.　*The root.*

GAULTHERIA.　　　　　Gaultheria procumbens.　*W.* II.
Partridge berry.　　　616.　*Bw.* II. 27.　*Bn.* I. 171.
　　　　　　　　　　　Folia.　*The leaves.*

GENTIANA CATESBÆI.　Gentiana Catesbæi.　*Elliott Bota-*
Blue gentian.　　　　*ny* I. 339.　*Bw.* II. 137.
　　　　　　　　　　　Radix.　*The root.*

GEUM.　　　　　　　　Geum rivale.　*W.* II. 1115.
Water avens.　　　　　Radix.　*The root.*

GRANATUM.　　　　　　Punica granatum.　*W.* II. 981.
Pomegranate.　　　　　Cortex fructus. *The rind of the fruit.*

HERACLEUM.　　　　　Heracleum lanatum.　*Mx.* I. 166.
Masterwort.　　　　　Radix.　*The root.*

IRIS FLORENTINA.　　Iris Florentina.　*W.* I. 236.
Florentine orris.　　Radix.　*The root.*

IRIS VERSICOLOR.　　Iris versicolor.　*W.* I. 233.　*Bw.*
Blue flag.　　　　　　I. 155.—Radix.　*The root.*

LACTUCA ELONGATA. Lactuca elongata. *W.* III. 1525.
Wild lettuce. Planta. *The plant.*

MAGNOLIA. Magnolia glauca. *W.* II. 1256.
Magnolia. *Bw.* II. 67. *Bn.* I. 77.
  Cortex. *The bark.* *Also the bark
  of Magnolia acuminata and M.
  tripetala.*

MARRUBIUM. Marrubium vulgare.
Horehound. Herba. *The herb.*

MENYANTHES. Menyanthes trifoliata. *W.* I. 811.
Buckbean. *Bw.* III. 55.—Radix. *The root.*

MONARDA. Monarda punctata. *W.* I. 126.
Monarda. Herba. *The herb.*

ORIGANUM. Origanum vulgare. *W.* III. 135.
Marjoram. Herba. *The herb.*

PETROSELINUM. Apium petroselinum. *W.* II. 1475.
Parsley. Planta. *The plant.*

PHYTOLACCÆ BACCÆ. Phytolacca decandra. *W.* II. 822.
Poke berries. Baccæ. *The berries.*

POLYGALA RUBELLA. Polygala rubella. *W.* III. 875. *Bw.*
Bitter polygala. III. 129.—Planta. *The plant.*

POLYPODIUM. Polypodium filix mas.
Polypody. Radix. *The root.*

PRINOS. Prinos verticillatus. *W.* II. 225.
Black alder. *Bw.* III. 141. *Bn.* I. 203.
  Cortex. *The bark.*

PRUNUS VIRGINIANA.   Prunus Virginiana. *W.* II. 985.
Wild cherry tree.   Cortex. *The bark.*

PYROLA.   Pyrola umbellata. *W.* II. 622. *Bw.*
Pyrola.   II. 15.
    Chimaphila umbellata. *Bn.* I. 17.
    Herba. *The herb.*

RANUNCULUS.   Ranunculus bulbosus. *W.* II. 1324.
Crowfoot.   *Bw.* III. 61.—Planta. *The plant.*

RHUS GLABRUM.   Rhus glabrum. *W.* I. 1478.
Sumach.   Baccæ. *The berries.*

RUBIA.   Rubia tinctorum. *W.* I. 603.
Madder.   Radix. *The root.*

RUBUS TRIVIALIS.   Rubus trivialis. *Mx.* I. 296.
Dewberry.   Cortex radicis. *The bark of the root.*

RUBUS VILLOSUS.   Rubus villosus. *W.* II. 1085. *Bw.*
Blackberry.   II. 160. *Bn.* II. 151.
    Cortex radicis. *The bark of the root.*

RUMEX BRITANNICA.   Rumex Britannica. *W.* II. 250.
Water dock.   Radix. *The root.*

RUMEX OBTUSIFOLIUS.   Rumex obtusifolius. *W.* II. 254.
Blunt leaved dock.   Radix. *The root.*

SAMBUCUS.   Sambucus Canadensis. *W.* I. 1494.
Elder.   Baccæ. *The berries.*

SANTALUM.   Pterocarpus santalinus. *W.* III.
Red sanders.   906.—Lignum. *The wood.*

SECALE CORNUTUM. *Spurred rye.* Called *Ergot.*	Secale cereale. *W.* I. 471. Clavus. *The spur.*
SESAMI OLEUM. *Benne oil.*	Sesamum orientale. *W.* III. 358. Oleum seminis. *The fixed oil of* *the seed.*
SOLIDAGO. *Golden rod.*	Solidago odora. *Bw.* I. 187. Folia. *The leaves.*
SPIRÆA. *Hardhack.*	Spiræa tomentosa. *W.* II. 1056. Radix. *The root.*
TANACETUM. *Tansy.*	Tanacetum vulgare. *W.* III. 1814. Herba. *The herb.*
TORMENTILLA. *Tormentil.*	Tormentilla erecta. *W.* II. 1112. Radix. *The root.*
TOXICODENDRON. *Poison oak.*	Rhus toxicodendron. *W.* I. 1481. Folia. *The leaves.*
TRIOSTEUM. *Fever root.*	Triosteum perfoliatum. *W.* I. 990. *Bw.* I. 90. *Bn.* I. 59. Radix. *The root.*
VERONICA. *Veronica.*	Veronica Virginica. *W.* I. 34. Radix. *The root.*
VIOLA. *Violet.*	Viola pedata. *W.* I. 1160. Planta. *The plant.*

8

PONDERA ET MENSURÆ.

AD quantitatem solidorum indicandam ponderum genere utimur, linguâ vernaculâ *Troy Weight* vocato, libramque sic dividimus, viz. :

Libra, ℔			Uncias duodecim	℥
Uncia	} habet {		Drachmas octo	ʒ
Drachma			Scrupulos tres	Ә
Scrupulus			Grana viginti.	g**r.**

Notas apposuimus quibus pondus quodque designare consuetum est.

Ad quantitatem liquidorum indicandam mensuris utimur ex congio vinario deductis, et quem ad usus medicinales sic dividimus, viz. :

Congius			Octantes octo	O
Octans	} habet {		Fluiduncias sedecim	f℥
Fluiduncia			Fluidrachmas octo	fʒ
Fluidrachma			Minima sexaginta	♏

Notas apposuimus quibus quamque mensuram designamus.

WEIGHTS AND MEASURES.

To express the quantity of solid bodies; we employ the kind of weight, which in common language is denominated *Troy Weight*, and divide the pound in the following manner.

The pound, ℔		Twelve ounces	℥
The ounce	contains	Eight drachms	ʒ
The drachm		Three scruples	Э
The scruple		Twenty grains	*gr.*

We have added the signs by which the several weights are denoted.

To express the quantity of liquids, we employ the measures which are derived from the wine gallon, and for medical purposes we divide it in the following manner.

The gallon, cong.		Eight pints	O
The pint	contains	Sixteen fluidounces	fℨ
The fluidounce		Eight fluidrachms	fʒ
The fluidrachm		Sixty minims	♍

We have added the signs by which we denote the several measures.

ACETA MEDICATA.

ACETUM OPII.

℞ Opii libram dimidiam.
    Aceti octantes tres.
    Myristicæ contusæ unciam unam, cum semisse.
    Croci unciam dimidiam.

Ad spissitudinem idoneam coque ; dein adde

    Sacchari uncias quatuor ;
    Cerevisiæ fermenti fluidunciam unam.

Digere per septem hebdomadas : dein coelo aperto, donec
fiat syrupus, expone. Denique effunde, cola, et vasis vitreis,
pauxillo sacchari unicuique vasi addito include.

ACETUM SCILLÆ.

℞ Scillæ siccatæ uncias duas.
    Aceti purificati octantes duos cum semisse.
    Alcoholis fluiduncias tres.

Macera scillam in aceto per decem dies, dein liquorem exprime, cui adde alcohol ; et, cum fæces subsederint, purum
effunde liquorem.

MEDICATED VINEGARS.

VINEGAR OF OPIUM.

COMMONLY CALLED BLACK DROP.

Take of Opium, half a pound.
   Vinegar, three pints.
   Nutmeg, bruised, one ounce and a half.
   Saffron, half an ounce.

Boil them to a proper consistence, then add

    Sugar, four ounces.
    Yeast, one fluid ounce.

Digest for seven weeks, then place in the open air until it becomes a syrup; lastly, decant, filter, and bottle it up, adding a little sugar to each bottle.

VINEGAR OF SQUILL.

Take of Squill, dried, two ounces.
   Purified vinegar, two pints and a half.
   Alcohol, three fluid ounces.

Macerate the squill in the vinegar for ten days; then press out the liquor, to which add the alcohol; and when the dregs have subsided, pour off the clear liquor.

ACIDA.

ACETUM DISTILLATUM.

℞ Aceti octantes octo.

Distillent in vasis vitreis aquæ balneo. Octante primo stil-
lato rejecto, octantes sex proximos serva.

ACETUM PURIFICATUM.

℞ Aceti congium unum.
   Carbonis ligni recentis, in pulverem redacti, unciam
   unam.

Carbonem aceto admisce, dein liquorem fervefac, despuma,
cola per laneum duplicem ; et postea, vel per chartam cola, vel,
dum subsideant fæces, relinque.

ACIDUM BENZOICUM.

℞ Benzoini quantumvis.

Liqua in retorta cervice lata, cui aptatus est excipulus non
lutulatus, et calore leni sublima : a tubo retortæ materiam subli-
matam, ne nimis accumuletur, remove subinde. Si oleo sit in-
quinata, inter chartæ bibulæ plicas involve ; dein fortiter preme,
et denuo sublima.

ACIDS.

DISTILLED VINEGAR.

Take of Vinegar, eight pints.

Distil in glass vessels, on a water bath. Throw away the first pint which comes over, and preserve the next six pints.

PURIFIED VINEGAR.

Take of Vinegar, one gallon.
Charcoal, fresh burnt and pulverized, one ounce.

Mix the charcoal and vinegar ; then bring the liquor to a boiling heat, skim, strain through double flannel, and afterwards filter through paper, or suffer the impurities to subside.

BENZOIC ACID.

Take of Benzoin, any quantity.

Liquify it in a wide necked retort, having a receiver fitted to it, but not luted, and sublime with a gentle heat. Remove the sublimed matter occasionally from the tube of the retort, lest it accumulate in too great quantity. If it be soiled with oil, wrap it between folds of blotting paper, then press it strongly, and repeat the sublimation.

ACIDUM CARBONICUM.

℞ Calcis carbonatis, in pulvere crasso quantumvis.

Huic superinfunde aquæ ad tegendum satis ; deinde adde paulatim acidum sulphuricum, donec non amplius elicitur aer.

ACIDUM CITRICUM.

℞ Limonum succi octantem unum.
Calcis carbonatis præparati unciam unam, seu, quan-
tum ad succum saturandum sit satis.
Acidi sulphurici diluti fluiduncias novem.

Calcis carbonatem succo fervefacto paulatim adde et agitando
misce ; deinde liquorem effunde. Citratem calcis remanentem,
aqua calida sæpius renovata, ablue ; deinde sicca. Pulveri sic-
cato adde acidum sulphuricum dilutum et per horæ partem sextam
coque : dein per linteum fortiter exprime ; et postea per chartam cola. Latex purus expressus, calore leni, vaporet, ut inter
frigescendum, fiant crystalli.

Ad crystallos puras reddendas, in aqua iterum atque tertium
solve ; et toties liquorem cola, decoque, et, dum fiant crystalli,
sepone.

ACIDUM SULPHURICUM DILUTUM.

℞ Acidi sulphurici fluidunciam unam.
Aquæ fluiduncias septem.

Misce paulatim.

CARBONIC ACID.

Take of Carbonate of lime, in coarse powder, any quantity.

Pour upon it so much water as shall completely cover it ; then add, by small quantities at a time, sulphuric acid until the gas ceases to be extricated.

CITRIC ACID.

Take of The juice of lemons, one pint.
Carbonate of lime prepared, one ounce, or as much as may be sufficient to saturate the juice.
Diluted sulphuric acid, nine fluid ounces.

Add the carbonate of lime by small portions at a time to the juice, whilst boiling, and mix it by stirring; then pour off the liquor. Wash the citrate of lime which remains by repeated additions of fresh warm water, and then dry it. Add the diluted sulphuric acid to the dried powder, and boil it for ten minutes ; then press it strongly through a linen cloth, and afterwards filter it through paper. Let the clear liquor which has passed be evaporated in a gentle heat, so that crystals may form as it gets cold.

To render these crystals pure, dissolve them a second and a third time in water, and after each solution filter the liquor, boil it down, and set it by to crystallize.

DILUTED SULPHURIC ACID.

Take of Sulphuric acid, one fluid ounce.
Water, seven fluid ounces.

Mix them gradually.

ACIDUM PRUSSICUM.

℞. Ferri Prussiatis uncias quatuor.
Hydrargyri nitrico-oxidi uncias duas cum semisse.
Aquæ distillatæ octantem unum.

Coque in vase vitreo, donec hydrargyri oxidum prorsus evanuerit ; liquorem cola ; et postea, colo superinfunde fluiduncias
tres aquæ calidæ distillatæ. Liquorem colatum retortæ vitreæ, cui cervix longa et tubulata est, infunde : et excipulus,
fluidunciam unam aquæ distillatæ continens, aptetur. Excipulo
sit tubus curvatus ad cyathum aquæ pertinens, ad hydrogenum
aera auferendum. In retortam per os tubulatum uncias duas
cum semisse ramentorum ferri purificatorum introducas ; et
postea, uncias duas acidi sulphurici. Excipulum, vel glacie,
vel aqua frigidissima circunda ; et a balneo arenæ unciæ tres,
sine bulliendo distillent.

ÆTHEREA.

ÆTHER SULPHURICUS.

℞. Alcholis.
Acidi sulphurici, singulorum libram cum semisse.

Alcohol retortæ vitreæ infunde, eique acidum paulatim adjice,
sæpius agitans, et cavens ne gradum centesimum vigesimum calor excedat, donec misceantur. Dein in arenam, ad gradum du-
centesimum prius calefactam, caute impone, ut quam celerrime
ebulliat liquor, transeatque æther in excipulum tubulatum, cui

PRUSSIC ACID.

Take of Prussiate of iron, four ounces.
  Nitric oxide of mercury, two ounces and a half.
  Distilled water, one pint.

Boil in a glass vessel until the oxide of mercury has wholly disappeared ; filter the solution, and afterwards pour upon the strainer three fluid ounces of hot distilled water. Put the filtered solution into a long necked and tubulated glass retort, and adapt a receiver containing one fluid ounce of distilled water. The receiver should have a bent tube extending from it to a cup of water, to carry off the hydrogen gas. Introduce two ounces of purified iron filings through the tubulure into the retort, and afterwards, two ounces (by weight) of sulphuric acid. Surround the receiver with ice, or very cold water, and distil without boiling, from a sand bath, three ounces.

PREPARATIONS OF ETHER.

SULPHURIC ETHER.

Take of Alcohol.
  Sulphuric acid each a pound and a half.

Pour the alcohol into a glass retort, then gradually add to it the acid, shaking it after each addition, and taking care that their temperature during the mixture do not exceed 120 Fahr. Immerse the retort very cautiously in a sand bath, previously heated to 200 so that the liquor may boil as speedily as possible,

aptatum est vas recipiens glacie vel aquâ refrigeratum. Distillet liquor, donec pars aliqua gravior transire incipiet, quæ sub æthere, in fundo receptaculi conspicitur. Liquori in retorta restanti rursus alcoholis uncias duodecim affunde, ut simili modo distillet æther.

OLEUM ÆTHEREUM.

Post distillationem ætheris sulphurici, lenito calore distillet iterum liquor, donec spuma nigra intumescat ; tum protinus ab igne retortam remove. Liquori qui restat in retortâ, aquam adjice, ut supernatet pars oleosa. Hanc aufer, eique admisce aquæ calcis quantum satis sit, ad acidum, quod inest, saturandum, et simul agita. Denique oleum æthereum separatum exime.

SPIRITUS ÆTHERIS SULPHURICI.

R. Ætheris sulphurici octantem dimidium.
   Alcoholis octantem unum.

Misce.

SPIRITUS ÆTHERIS SULPHURICI COMPOSITUS.

R. Spiritus ætheris sulphurici octantem unum.
   Olei ætherei fluidrachmas duas.

Misce.

and let the ether pass over into a tubulated receiver, to the tubulure of which another receiver is applied, which is to be kept cold by immersion in ice or water   Distil the liquor until the heavier part also begins to pass over and appear under the ether in the bottom of the receiver.   To the liquor which remains in the retort, pour on one pint more of alcohol, and repeat the distillation in the same manner.

ETHEREAL OIL.

After the distillation of sulphuric ether, carry on the distillation with a less degree of heat until a black froth begins to rise : then immediately remove the retort from the fire.   Add sufficient water to the liquor in the retort, that the oily parts may float upon the surface.   Separate this and add to it as much lime water as may be necessary to neutralize the adherent acid, and shake them together.   Lastly collect the ethereal oil which separates.

SPIRIT OF SULPHURIC ETHER.

Take of Sulphuric ether half a pint.
        Alcohol one pint.

Mix.

COMPOUND SPIRIT OF SULPHURIC ETHER.

FORMERLY HOFFMAN'S ANODYNE LIQUOR.

Take of Spirit of sulphuric ether one pint.
        Ethereal oil two fluid drachms.

Mix.

SPIRITUS ÆTHERIS NITROSI.

R. Alcoholis octantes duos.
Acidi nitrici, uncias tres.

Alcoholi acidum paulatim adjice, et misce, cavens ne gradum
centesimum vigesimum calor excedat : tum leni calore, distillent
fluidunciæ viginti quatuor.

ALCOHOL.

ALCOHOL DILUTUM.

R. Alcoholis octantem unum.
Aquæ distillatæ octantem unum.

Misce.

ALUMEN.

ALUMEN EXSICCATUM.

R. Aluminis quantumvis.

In vase vel fictili vel ferreo super igne liquescat, et cum cessaverit ebullitio, remove.

SPIRIT OF NITROUS ETHER.

Take of Alcohol two pints.
Nitric acid, three ounces.

Mix them very gradually together by pouring the acid into the alcohol, and taking care that the heat during the mixture does not exceed 120. Then, by means of a gentle heat, distil twenty-four fluid ounces.

ALCOHOL.

DILUTED ALCOHOL.

Take of Alcohol, one pint.
Distilled water, one pint.

Mix.

ALUM.

DRIED ALUM.

Take of Alum, any quantity.

Melt it in an earthen or iron vessel over the fire, and remove it when it ceases to boil.

AMMONIA.

ALCOHOL AMMONIATUM.

℞. Alcoholis octantes duos.
Calcis recentis libram unam.
Ammoniæ muriatis in pulverem redacti uncias octo.
Aquæ octantem dimidium.

Calci adjice aquam, et, dum calx macerando dilabitur, sepone ;
dein calcem intromitte in retortam vitream arenæ balneo superimpositam, cujus cervici aptatus est excipulus, qui frigidus servandus est ; calci immitte ammoniæ muriatem et alcohol, et
lento igni distillent, donec liquor in excipulo ad octantem cum
semisse creverit.

AMMONIÆ ACETAS LIQUIDUS.

℞. Ammoniæ carbonatis, in pulverem redacti quantumvis.

Adde paulatim et sæpe agitando, aceti purificati quantum ad
saturandum accurate ammoniæ carbonatem suffecerit.

AQUA AMMONIÆ.

℞. Ammoniæ muriatis in pulverem redacti libram unam.
Calcis recentis libram unam cum semisse.
Aquæ congium unum.

Calci adjice aquæ octantes duos et dum calx macerando dilabitur sepone : dein calcem intromitte in retortam vitream arenæ

AMMONIA.

AMMONIATED ALCOHOL.

Take of Alcohol, two pints.
Lime, recently burnt, one pound.
Muriate of ammonia, in powder, eight ounces.
Water, half a pint.

Add the water to the lime, let them stand till the lime is slacked ; then put the lime into a glass retort resting on a sand bath, to the beak of which is connected a glass receiver, which is to be kept cold : add to the lime the muriate of ammonia and the alcohol, and distil with a slow fire until the liquid in the receiver amounts to one pint and a half.

LIQUID ACETATE OF AMMONIA.
COMMONLY CALLED SPIRIT OF MINDERERUS.

Take of Carbonate of ammonia, in powder, any quantity.

Add, by small portions, with frequent agitation, so much purified vinegar, as shall be sufficient exactly to saturate the carbonate of ammonia.

WATER OF AMMONIA.

Take of Muriate of ammonia, in powder, one pound.
Lime, fresh burnt, one pound and a half.
Water, one gallon.

Add to the lime, two pints of the water ; let them stand until the lime is slacked, then put the lime into a glass retort, resting

10

balneo superimpositam, cujus cervici aptatus est excipulus amplus qui frigidus servandus est. Calci ammoniæ muriatem et aquam restantem adde, et igne leni distillent, donec liquor in excipulo ad octantes duos creverit.

AMMONIÆ CARBONAS.

℞. Ammoniæ muriatis libram unam.
Calcis carbonatis mollis siccati libram unam cum semisse.

In pulverem separatim redige dein assidue permisce ; et ex rétorta, in excipulum frigidum sublima.

AQUA AMMONIÆ CARBONATIS.

℞. Ammoniæ muriatis.
Potassæ carbonatis, utriusque uncias sexdecim
Aquæ octantes duos.

Salibus mistis, et retortæ vitreæ intromissis, aquam infunde, et in arenæ balneo, calore gradatim aucto, ad siccitatem fiat distillatio.

AMMONIÆ HYDROSULPHURETUM.

℞. Aquæ ammoniæ fliduncias quatuor.
In apparatu chemico, subjice rivo aërio qui oriatur ex

Antimonii sulphureti unciis quatuor.
Acidi muriatici unciis octo, prius aquæ octantibus duobus cum semisse dilutis.

Quod exinde oriatur, in vase vitreo, accurate obturato, servetur.

on a sand bath, to the beak of which is connected a large glass receiver, which is to be kept cold ; add to the lime the muriate of ammonia, and the remainder of the water ; and distil with a slow fire, until the liquid in the receiver amount to two pints.

CARBONATE OF AMMONIA.

Take of Muriate of ammonia, one pound.
   Soft carbonate of lime, dried, one pound and a half.

Having triturated them separately, mix them thoroughly, and sublime from a retort into a receiver kept cold.

WATER OF CARBONATE OF AMMONIA.

Take of Muriate of ammonia ;
   Carbonate of potass, each sixteen ounces.
   Water, two pints.

Having mixed the salts and put them into a glass retort, pour the water upon them, and distil to dryness in a sand bath, gradually increasing the heat.

HYDROSULPHURET OF AMMONIA.

Take of Water of ammonia, four fluid ounces ;

Subject it in a chemical apparatus to a stream of the gas, which arises from

   Sulphuret of antimony, four ounces.
   Muriatic acid, eight ounces, previously diluted with
    two pints and a half of water.

Preserve the product in a close stopped glass vessel.

ANTIMONIUM.

PULVIS ANTIMONIALIS.

℞. Antimonii sulphureti, in pulverem crassum triti, partem unam.
Cornu cervi rasi, partes duas.

Misce, et in ollam ferream latam injice, igne rubentem, et assidue agita, donec in materiam coloris cinerei usta fuerint, quam ab igne aufer, et in pulverem tere, et crucibulo loricato immitte ; huic crucibulum aliud inversum, cui parvum sit in fundo foramen, luto conjunge, ignemque subministra, quem ad calorem candentem sensim auge, et ita auctum serva per horas duas ; denique materiam frigefactam in pulverem subtilissimum tere.

ANTIMONII MURIAS.

℞. Antimonii oxidi ;
Acidi sulphurici, utriusque libram unam.
Sodae muriatis exsiccati libras duas.

Acidum sulphuricum retortae infunde, paulatim addens sodae muriatem et antimonii oxidum, prius commista ; dein super arenam calidam fiat distillatio. Materia distillata per aliquot dies aëri pateat, ut liquescat ; tum effundatur è faecibus pars liquida.

ANTIMONY.

ANTIMONIAL POWDER.

CALLED JAMES POWDER.

Take of Sulphuret of antimony, in coarse powder, one part.
Hartshorn, in shavings, two parts.

Mix and put them in a wide, red hot iron pot, and stir the mixture constantly, until it be burnt into a matter of an ash grey colour, which is to be then removed from the fire, ground into powder, and put into a coated crucible; lute to this crucible another inverted over it, and perforated in the bottom with a small hole, and apply the fire, which is to be raised gradually to a white heat, and kept in that increased state for two hours; lastly, grind the matter, when cold, into a very fine powder.

MURIATE OF ANTIMONY.

Take of Oxide of antimony;
Sulphuric acid, of each, one pound.
Dried muriate of soda, two pounds.

Pour the sulphuric acid into a retort, gradually adding the muriate of soda, and oxide of antimony, previously mixed. Then perform the distillation in a sand bath. Expose the distilled matter for several days to the air, that it may deliquesce, and then pour the liquor from the feces.

ANTIMONII OXIDUM.

℞. Antimonii sulphureti ;
    Potassæ nitratis, utriusque pondera paria.

Separatim trita, et bene commista injiciantur in crucibulum candens. Peracta deflagratione, materia rubescens a crusta albicante separetur, et teratur in pulverem, qui sæpius lavetur aquâ calidâ, donec hæc insipida maneat.

ANTIMONII OXIDUM VITRIFICATUM.

℞. Antimonii sulphureti, quantumvis, in pulverem crassum, arenæ instar, contriti.

Insterne super vas fictile, non vitreatum, parum profundum, ignemque suppone lenem, ut antimonii sulphuretum lente calefiat ; pulverem interea assidue agitans, ne in grumos coëat. Vapores albi, sulphur olentes, ex eo orientur. Cùm hi, eodem calore deficiant, ignem auge aliquantum, ut iterum vapores exhalet ; et sic perge, donec pulvis igne tandem rubescens vapores non amplius exhalet. Pulvis ille crucibulo inditus liquescat igne violento, donec vitri liquefacti speciem induat; dein effundatur super laminam äeneam calefactam.

ANTIMONII OXIDUM VITRIFICATUM CUM CERA.

℞. Ceræ flavæ, partem unam.
    Antimonii oxidi vitrificati, partes octo.

OXIDE OF ANTIMONY.

FORMERLY CROCUS OF ANTIMONY.

Take of Sulphuret of antimony ;
　　Nitrate of potass, of each equal weights.

After they are separately powdered and well mixed, let them
be thrown into a red hot crucible. When the deflagration is
over, separate the reddish matter from the whitish crust, and
reduce it to a powder, which is to be repeatedly washed with
hot water, till the water remains insipid.

VITRIFIED OXIDE OF ANTIMONY.

FORMERLY GLASS OF ANTIMONY.

Take of Sulphuret of antimony, any quantity, beat into coarse
　　powder like sand.

Strew it upon an unglazed shallow earthern vessel, and place
it over a gentle fire, that the sulphuret of antimony may be slowly heated, at the same time stirring the powder constantly, to
prevent it from running into lumps. White vapours, having the
odour of sulphur, will arise from it. When these cease with
the degree of heat first applied, raise the heat a little, so that
the vapours may arise again ; go on in this manner, till the
powder, brought to a red heat, exhales no more vapours. Melt
this powder in a crucible, with an intense heat, till it assumes
the appearance of melted glass ; then pour it upon a heated
brass plate.

VITRIFIED OXIDE OF ANTIMONY WITH WAX.

FORMERLY CERATED GLASS OF ANTIMONY.

Take of Yellow wax, one part.
　　Vitrified oxide of antimony, eight parts.

Ceræ in vase ferreo liquifactæ injice oxidum in pulverem tritum, et torre, igne leni, per horæ quadrantem, spathulâ assidue agitans ; dein effunde materiam, quæ frigefacta teratur in pulverem.

ANTIMONII SULPHURETUM PRÆCIPITATUM.

℞. Aquæ potassæ, libras quatuor.
Aquæ octantes tres.
Antimonii sulphureti præparati, libras duas.

Coque in olla ferrea operta, super ignem lenem, per horas tres, sæpe agitans spathulâ ferreâ, et addens aquam prout opus fuerit. Liquorem calidum cola per linteum duplex, et colato adde acidi sulphurici diluti quantum satis sit ad dejiciendum sulphuretum, aquâ calidâ diligenter lavandum.

ANTIMONII SULPHURETUM PRÆPARATUM.

Antimonii sulphuretum præparatur eodum modum ac calcis carbonas.

ANTIMONIUM TARTARIZATUM.

℞. Antimonii in pulverem redacti partem unam.
Acidi sulphurici partes duas.

Melt the wax in an iron vessel, and throw into it the powdered oxide ; roast the mixture over a gentle fire, for a quarter of an hour, continually stirring it with a spatula ; then pour it out, and, when cold, grind it into powder.

PRECIPITATED SULPHURET OF ANTIMONY.

FORMERLY GOLDEN SULPHUR OF ANTIMONY.

Take of Solution of potass, four pounds.
   Water, three pints.
   Prepared sulphuret of antimony, two pounds.

Boil them in a covered iron pot, over a slow fire, for three hours, frequently stirring the mixture with an iron spatula, and adding water as it may be required. Strain the hot liquor through a double linen cloth, and add to it, when strained, as much diluted sulphuric acid as may be necessary to precipitate the sulphuret, which must be well washed with warm water.

PREPARED SULPHURET OF ANTIMONY.

Sulphuret of antimony is prepared in the same way as carbonate of lime.

TARTARIZED ANTIMONY.

FORMERLY TARTAR EMETIC.

Take of Antimony, (the metal) in powder, one part.
   Sulphuric acid, two parts.

11

In vase ferreo, aperto, ad siccitatem, spathula ferrea sæpe mixturam agitans, coque. Acidum adhuc liberum aqua ablue ; et residuum sicca ; cui potassæ supertartratem pari pondere, in aqua solutum adde. Dein in vase ferreo coque, cola, et, dum fiant crystalli, sepone. Liquor, qui restat, si iterum vaporatus et colatus, crystallos iterum deponet ; si autem hæ minus lucidæ sint, denuo solvantur et deponantur.

AQUÆ MEDICATÆ.

AQUA ACIDI CARBONICI.

℞. Aquæ quantumvis.

Huic, antliâ condensanti, tantum acidi carbonici ingere, quantum volumen suum decies circiter superat.

AQUA MAGNESIÆ.

℞. Aquæ congium unum.
Magnesiæ carbonatis drachmas tres.

Misce, et antliâ condensanti, tantum acidi carbonici ingere, quantum volumen suum decies circiter superat.

Hoc modo parantur

AQUA POTASSÆ,

Ex potassæ subcarbonatis uncia una.

AQUA SODÆ.

Ex sodæ subcarbonatis unciis duabus.

Boil them to dryness in an open iron vessel, frequently stirring the mixture with an iron spatula. Wash out all the uncombined acid, with water, and dry the residuum; to which add an equal weight of supertartrate of potass, dissolved in water; then boil in an iron vessel, filter, and set by to crystallize. The evaporation, filtration, and crystallization may be repeated with the fluid which remains; but if the crystals are not perfectly clear, they must be dissolved in water and recrystallized.

MEDICATED WATERS.

CARBONIC ACID WATER.
COMMONLY CALLED SELTZER WATER.

Take of Water, any quantity.

Impregnate it with about ten times its volume of carbonic acid gas, by means of a forcing pump.

MAGNESIA WATER.
COMMONLY CALLED LIQUID MAGNESIA.

Take of Water, one gallon.
Carbonate of magnesia, three drachms.

Mix, and impregnate it with about ten times its volume of carbonic acid gas, by means of a forcing pump.

In like manner are prepared
POTASS WATER,

From one ounce of subcarbonate of potass.

SODA WATER,

From two ounces of subcarbonate of soda.

AQUÆ DISTILLATÆ.

AQUA AURANTII CORTICIS.

℞. Aurantii corticis recentis libras duas.

His effundatur aquæ satis ad evitandum empyreuma. Post macerationem debitam distillentur octantes decem.

Hoc modo parantur
AQUA CINNAMOMI,
Ex cinnamomi contusi librâ unâ.

AQUA MENTHÆ PIPERITÆ,
Ex menthæ piperitæ florentis libris tribus.

AQUA MENTHÆ VIRIDIS,
Ex menthæ viridis florentis libris tribus.

AQUA ROSARUM,
Ex rosarum recentium libris sex.

Singulis harum aquarum octantibus adde alcoholis diluti fluidunciam dimidiam.

Aquæ distillatæ in lagenis vitreis obturatis serventur.

AQUA DISTILLATA.

Aqua distilletur vasis permundis, donec ejus duo circiter trientes stillaverint. Aquam distillatam in lagena vitrea servato.

DISTILLED WATERS.

WATER OF ORANGE PEEL.

Take of Fresh orange peel, two pounds.

Pour upon it water enough to prevent empyreuma, and after due maceration distil ten pints.

In the same manner are prepared
CINNAMON WATER,

From a pound of bruised cinnamon.

PEPPERMINT WATER,

From three pounds of peppermint in flower.

SPEARMINT WATER,

From three pounds of spearmint in flower.

ROSE WATER,

From six pounds of fresh roses.

To every pint of distilled water add half a fluidounce of diluted alcohol.

Distilled waters should be kept in well stopped glass bottles.

DISTILLED WATER.

Let water be distilled in very clean vessels until about two thirds have come over, which is to be kept in a glass bottle.

12

ARGENTUM.

ARGENTI NITRAS.

R. Argenti puri, in laminas complanati, et minutatim
consecti, unciam unam.
Acidi nitrici fluidunciam unam.
Aquæ distillatæ fluiduncias duas.

Acidum cum aqua misce, et in ea mistura, arenæ balneo, argentum solve. Dein calorem gradatim auge, ut argenti nitras sic-
cetur. Salem crucibulo, leni super igni solve, donec, aqua expulsa, cessaverit ebullitio, et instar olei fluxerit massa. Tum
cito in formas idoneas effunde. Denique, in vase vitreo, accurate obturato, et a luce remoto, serva.

ARSENICUM.

LIQUOR POTASSÆ ARSENIATIS.

R. Acidi arseniosi, in pulverem subtilem redacti ;
Potassæ subcarbonatis, utriusque grana sexaginta
quatuor.
Aquæ distillatæ octantem unum.

In vase vitreo concoque donec acidum arseniosum omne re-
solvatur. Liquorem frigefactum in mensuram octariam infunde ;
et adde

Alcoholis fluidrachmas quatuor,

Et aquæ distillatæ quantum suffecerit ad mensuram complen-
dam.

SILVER.

NITRATE OF SILVER.
FORMERLY LUNAR CAUSTIC.

Take of Pure silver, flattened into plates, and cut into pieces,
one ounce.
Nitric acid, one fluidounce.
Distilled water, two fluidounces.

Mix the nitric acid and water, and dissolve the silver therein
on a sand bath; then increase the heat gradually that the nitrate of silver may be dried. Melt the salt in a crucible over a
slow fire, until the water being evaporated, it ceases to boil, and
the mass flows like oil; then pour it quickly into moulds of convenient shape. Lastly, keep it in a glass vessel very well
stopped, and secured from light.

ARSENIC.

ARSENICAL SOLUTION.

Take of Arsenious acid, in fine powder;
Subcarbonate of potass, each sixty-four grains.
Distilled water, one pint.

Boil them together in a glass vessel until the arsenic is entirely dissolved. When the solution is cold, pour it into a pint
measure, and add thereto

Alcohol, four fluidrachms,

And so much distilled water, as shall fill up the measure.

AURUM.

AURI MURIAS.

R. Auri quantumvis.

Calore leni solve in mistura, ex acidi nitrici parte una, et acidi muriatici partibus duabus composita ; tum liquor ad siccitatem leni calore vaporet. Adde residuo sodæ muriatis pondus par, et assidue permisce. Misturam in aqua distillata solve, et ad siccitatem paulatim vaporet. Massam collectam serva in vase vitreo accurate vitro obturato, et a luce submoto.

BARYTA.

BARYTÆ MURIAS.

R. Barytæ sulphatis, libras duas.
  Carbonis ligni, in pulverem triti, uncias quatuor.

Igne torreatur sulphas, quò facilius teratur in pulverem tenuissimum, cui bene admiscendus est pulvis carbonatis ligni. Indatur materies crucibulo, et, adaptato operculo, urgeatur igne forti per horas sex Materia bene trita immittatur in aquæ bullientis octantes sex in vase vitreo vel figulino, et agitatione permisceatur, aëris aditu, quantum fieri possit, occluso.

Stet vas in balneo vaporis, donec subsederit pars non soluta ; dein effundatur liquor. Illi affundantur denuo aquæ bullientis octantes quatuor ; quæ post agitationem et subsidentiam priori

GOLD.

MURIATE OF GOLD.

Take of Pure gold, any quantity.

Dissolve it by means of a moderate heat, in a mixture formed by uniting one part of nitric acid with two parts of muriatic acid ; evaporate the solution to dryness by a gentle heat ; add to the residuum an equal weight of muriate of soda, and mix them thoroughly together. Dissolve the mixture in distilled water, and evaporate slowly to dryness. Collect the mass and keep it in a glass-stopped phial, which should be accurately closed, and preserved from the action of light.

BARYTA.

MURIATE OF BARYTA.

Take of Sulphate of baryta, two pounds.
Charcoal in powder, four ounces.

Roast the sulphate, that it may be more easily reduced to a very fine powder, with which the powdered charcoal is to be intimately mixed. Put the mixture into a crucible, and having fitted it with a cover, heat it with a strong fire for six hours. Then triturate the matter well, and throw it into six pints of water in an earthen or glass vessel, and mix them by agitation, preventing as much as possible the action of the air.

Let the vessel stand in a vapour bath until the part not dissolved shall subside, then pour off the liquor. On the undissolved part pour four pints more of boiling water, which, after agitation, and deposition, are to be added to the former liquor.

liquori addantur. Liquori adhuc calido, vel si friguerit iterum
calefacto, instilletur acidum muriaticum, quandiu moverit effervescentiam.   Dein coletur, et vaporet ut crystalli formentur.

LIQUOR BARYTÆ MURIATIS.

℞. Barytæ muriatis unciam unam.
   Aquæ distillatæ fluidunciam tres.

Solve.

BISMUTHUM.

BISMUTHI SUBNITRAS.

℞. Bismuthi unciam unam.
   Acidi nitrici ;
   Aquæ, utriusque fluiduncias tres.

Acidum nitricum aquæ agitando admisce ; tum bismuthum,
mortario ferreo in pulverem subactum acido diluto gradatim
adde ; et vas, donec solutum fuerit metallum, sepone. Liquorem purum in vas vitreum amplum transfunde, et congium
dimidium aquæ distillatæ liquoris fluidunciæ unicuique infunde.
Cum præcipitatum album subsederit, liquidum supernatans effunde ; et additionem et transfusionem, donec aqua insipida
evadet, itera   Pulverem albidum collectum, calore nullo adhibito, sicca ; et in vase vitreo, luce exclusâ, serva.

Into the liquor, when still warm, or if it shall have cooled, again heated, drop muriatic acid as long as it excites any effervescence. Then strain it, and evaporate it so as to crystallize.

SOLUTION OF MURIATE OF BARYTA.

Take of Muriate of baryta, one ounce.
Distilled water, three fluidounces.

Dissolve.

BISMUTH.

SUB-NITRATE OF BISMUTH.

FORMERLY WHITE OXIDE OF BISMUTH.

Take of Bismuth, one ounce.
Nitric acid ;
Water, each three fluidounces.

Add the water and nitric acid together with agitation, then reduce the bismuth to powder in an iron mortar. Add it by small portions at a time to the diluted acid, and allow the vessel to remain at rest, until the metal is dissolved. Decant the clear solution into a large glass vessel, and for every fluidounce of the liquid, pour in half a gallon of distilled water. When the white precipitate has subsided, pour off the supernatant liquid, and repeat the addition and decantation until the water comes off tasteless ; collect the white powder, dry it without the application of heat, and keep it in a glass vessel secluded from light.

CALX.

AQUA CALCIS.

R. Calcis selibram.
Aquæ distillatæ ferventis octantes duodecim.

Calci aquam affunde, et simul agita ; tum protinus vas contege, et sepone per horas tres ; dein liquorem cum calce superstite in vasis vitreis obturatis serva, et, quandocunque utendum est, ex limpido liquore sume.

CALCIS CARBONAS PRÆPARATUS.

R. Calcis carbonatis mollis libram unam.

Calcis carbonati adjice aquæ paululum, et tere, ut fiat pulvis subtilis. Hunc in vas amplum aquâ plenum conjice ; tum agita, et, brevi morâ interpositâ, in vas aliud aquam adhuc turbidam supernatantem transmitte, et sepone, dum subsidat pulvis ; denique, rejectâ aquâ, pulverem exsicca.

LIQUOR CALCIS MURIATIS.

R. Calcis carbonatis durioris, in frusta contusi, uncias novem.
Acidi muriatici uncias sexdecim.
Aquæ octantem dimidium.

Acidum cum aqua, misce, et frusta calcis carbonatis paulatim adde. Effervescentiâ finitâ, digere per horam ; liquorem effunde, et per vaporationem ad siccitatem redige. Residuum solve in sesquialtero pondere aquæ ; et demum cola.

LIME.

LIME WATER.

Take of Lime, half a pound.
Boiling water, twelve pints.

Pour the water upon the lime and stir them together ; next cover the vessel immediately, and let it stand for three hours ; then keep the solution upon the remaining lime in stopped glass bottles, and pour off the clear liquor when it is wanted for use

PREPARED CARBONATE OF LIME.

Take of Soft carbonate of lime, one pound.

Add a small quantity of water to the carbonate of lime, and grind it into a fine powder ; throw this powder into a large vessel full of water, then stir it, and after a short interval, pour the supernatant turbid solution into another vessel, and set it by, that the powder may subside ; lastly, having poured away the water, dry the powder.

SOLUTION OF MURIATE OF LIME.

Take of Hard carbonate of lime, broken in pieces, nine ounces.
Muriatic acid, sixteen ounces.
Water, half a pint.

Mix the acid with the water, and gradually add the pieces of lime. When the effervescence has ceased, digest them for an hour, pour off the liquor, and evaporate to dryness. Dissolve the residuum in its weight and a half of water, and, lastly, filter the solution.

CERATA.

———

Cerata parantur ex oleo vel adipe cum cerâ et resinâ in unum corpus redacto, quibus medicamenta varia sæpe commiscentur. Crassitudinem talem habere debent, ut in linamentum vel linteolum facile obducantur ; sed ut non diffluant cum corpori apponantur.

———

CERATUM ARSENICI.

℞. Cerati simplicis unciam unam.
Acidi arseniosi in pulverem triti scrupulum unum.

Cerato igne emollito adjice acidum et misce.

———

CERATUM CANTHARIDUM.

℞. Ceræ flavæ ;
Resinæ pini ;
Olei olivæ singulorum partes duas.
Cantharidum in pulverem tritarum partes tres.

Ceræ, resinæ et oleo prius simul liquefactis cantharides adjice, et assidue move donec refrixerint.

———

CERATUM JUNIPERI VIRGINIANI.

℞. Cerati resinosi partes sex.
Juniperi Virginiani in pulverem triti partem unam.

Cerato igne lento emollito juniperum adjice et misce.

CERATES.

———

Cerates are composed of oil or lard united with wax and resin, to which various medicaments are frequently added. They should be of such consistence that they may be easily spread on lint or linen, yet not melt or run when applied to the body.

———

CERATE OF ARSENIC.

Take of Simple cerate, one ounce.
Arsenious acid in powder, one scruple.

Soften the cerate, and mix in the acid.

———

CERATE OF CANTHARIDES.

Take of Yellow wax ;
Pine resin ;
Olive oil, each, two parts.
Cantharides in powder, three parts.

To the wax, resin and oil, previously melted together, add the cantharides, carefully stirring the whole until cool.

———

CERATE OF RED CEDAR.

Take of Resin cerate, six parts.
Red cedar in powder, one part.

To the cerate previously softened, add the cedar and mix.

CERATUM PLUMBI SUBACETATIS LIQUIDI.

R. Plumbi subacetatis liquidi fluiduncias duas cum se-
misse.
Ceræ flavæ uncias quatuor.
Olei olivæ fluiduncias novem.
Camphoræ drachmam dimidiam.

Ceram liquefactam cum olei fluidunciis octo misce : tum ab
igne remove, et ubi primum lentescant liquorem plumbi subacetatis paulatim adjice, et assidue move spatha lignea donec refrixerint. Denique cum his camphoram in reliquo oleo liquatam
misce.

CERATUM PLUMBI SUBCARBONATIS COMPOSI-
TUM.

R. Emplastri plumbi subcarbonatis compositi partes
quinque.
Olei olivæ partem unam.

Emplastro liquefacto adjice oleum, assidue movens donec refrixerint.

CERATUM RESINOSUM.

R. Adipis partes octo.
Resinæ pini partes quinque.
Ceræ flavæ partes duas.

Liquefac simul et assidue move donec refrixerint.

CERATE WITH SUBACETATE OF LEAD.

GOULARD'S CERATE.

Take of Liquid subacetate of lead two fluidounces and a half.
    Yellow wax, four ounces.
    Olive oil, nine fluidounces.
    Camphor, half a drachm.

Mix the wax, previously melted, with eight ounces of oil : remove the mixture from the fire, and when it begins to thicken, gradually pour in the liquid subacetate of lead, stirring constantly with a wooden spatula until cool. Lastly, add the camphor dissolved in the remainder of the oil, and mix.

CERATE OF SUBCARBONATE OF LEAD.

Take of Compound plaster of subcarbonate of lead, five parts.
    Olive oil, one part.

To the plaster, previously melted, add the oil, stirring the whole constantly together until cool.

RESIN CERATE.

Take of Lard, eight parts.
    Pine resin, five parts.
    Yellow wax, two parts.

Melt and stir them together until cool.

13

CERATUM RESINOSUM COMPOSITUM.

℞. Sevi ;
　　Ceræ flavæ utriusque libram unam.
　　Resinæ pini libram unam.
　　Terebinthinæ libram dimidiam.
　　Lini olei octantem dimidiam.

Liquefac simul, et per linteum exprime.

———

CERATUM SABINÆ.

℞. Cerati resinosi partes sex.
　　Sabinæ foliorum in pulverem tritorum partem unam.

Cerato emollito sabinam adjice, et misce.

———

CERATUM SAPONIS.

℞. Saponis uncias octo.
　　Ceræ flavæ uncias decem.
　　Plumbi oxidi semivitrei in pulverem triti libram unam.
　　Olei olivæ octantem unam.
　　Aceti congium unum.

Coque acetum cum plumbi oxido, lento igne, assidue movens, donec in unum coëant ; dein adjice saponem et iterum simili modo coque, donec humor penitus consumptus fuerit ; denique ceram cum oleo prius liquefactam cæteris immisce.

COMPOUND RESIN CERATE.

Take of Suet ;
        Yellow wax, each, one pound.
        Pine resin, one pound.
        Turpentine, half a pound.
        Flax seed oil half a pint.

Melt them together, and strain through linen.

SAVIN CERATE.

Take of Resin cerate, six parts.
        Savin leaves, in powder, one part.

To the cerate, previously softened, add the savin and mix.

SOAP CERATE.

Take of Castile soap, eight ounces.
        Yellow wax, ten ounces.
        Semivitreous oxide of lead, in powder, one pound.
        Olive oil, a pint.
        Vinegar, a gallon.

Boil the vinegar with the oxide of lead, over a slow fire, constantly stirring until the union is complete ; then add the soap and boil it again in a similar manner, until the liquid part is evaporated ; then mix in the wax, previously melted with the oil.

CERATUM SIMPLEX.

℞. Olei olivæ partes sex.
Ceræ albæ partes tres.
Spermatis ceti partem unam.

Spermati ceti et ceræ simul liquefactis oleum adjice, et move donec refrixerint.

CERATUM ZINCI CARBONATIS IMPURI.

℞. Adipis libram unam.
Ceræ flavæ uncias quinque cum semisse.
Zinci carbonatis impuri libram dimidiam.

Ceræ et adipi simul liquefactis zincum adjice et assidue move donec refrixerint.

COLLYRIA.

COLLYRIUM PLUMBI ACETATIS.

℞. Plumbi acetatis scrupulum unum.
Aquæ distillatæ octantem dimidium.

Fiat solutio.

COLLYRIUM PLUMBI ACETATIS ET OPII.

℞. Plumbi acetatis scrupulum unum.
Aquæ distillatæ octantem dimidium.
Tincturæ opii fluidrachmam unam.

Misce.

SIMPLE CERATE.

Take of Olive oil, six parts.
    White wax, three parts.
    Spermaceti, one part.

Melt the wax and spermaceti together, then add the oil, stirring until the whole is cool.

CERATE OF IMPURE CARBONATE OF ZINC,
TURNER'S CERATE.

Take of Lard, one pound.
    Yellow wax, five ounces and a half.
    Impure carbonate of zinc, half a pound.

To the lard and wax, previously melted together, add the zinc, carefully stirring the whole until cool.

COLLYRIA.

COLLYRIUM OF ACETATE OF LEAD.

Take of Acetate of lead, a scruple.
    Distilled water, half a pint.

Mix and dissolve.

COLLYRIUM OF OPIUM AND ACETATE OF LEAD.

Take of Acetate of lead, a scruple.
    Distilled water, half a pint.
    Tincture of opium, a fluidrachm.
Mix.

COLLYRIUM ZINCI ACETATIS.

R. Zinci sulphatis grana duodecim.
Plumbi acetatis grana sexdecim.
Aquæ distillatæ octantem dimidium.

Fiat solutio, et precipitatione facto, effundatur liquor purus.

COLLYRIUM ZINCI SULPHATIS.

R. Zinci sulphatis grana duodecim.
Aquæ distillatæ octantem dimidium.

Fiat solutio.

CONFECTIONES.

Confectio massa composita est ex medicamento quovis cum saccharino tali modo confecta, ut vel virtutes conservet, vel saporem obteget, vel facilius adhibendum reddat.

CONFECTIO AROMATICA.

R. Lauri cassiæ corticis ;
Cardamomi ;
Zingiberis, singulorum unciam unam.

In pulverem subtilissimum subige, et adde

Syrupi aurantii corticis fluiduncias sex.

Misce, et diligenter contunde.

COLLYRIUM OF ACETATE OF ZINC.

Take of Sulphate of zinc twelve grains.
          Acetate of lead, sixteen grains.
          Distilled water, half a pint.

Mix and dissolve, and after precipitation pour off the clear liquid.

———

COLLYRIUM OF SULPHATE OF ZINC.

Take of Sulphate of zinc twelve grains.
          Distilled water, half a pint.

Mix and dissolve.

———

CONFECTIONS.

———

A confection is a compound mass, prepared by uniting a medicinal substance with saccharine matter, in such manner as to preserve the virtues of the medicament, to cover its taste, or to facilitate its administration.*

———

AROMATIC CONFECTION.

Take of Cassia bark ;
          Cardamom ;
          Ginger, of each, one ounce.
Reduce them to a very fine powder, and add
          Syrup of orange peel, six fluidounces.
Mix, and beat them well together.

———

* Under this head are included the Conserves, Electuaries, and Confections of former Pharmacopœias.

CONFECTIO AURANTII CORTICIS.

℞. Aurantii corticis recentis partem unam.
Sacchari partes tres.

Aurantii corticem, adjuto paulatim saccharo, in pulpam contunde.

CONFECTIO CASSIÆ.

℞. Cassiæ fistulæ pulpæ partes quatuor.
Tamarindi pulpæ ;
Mannæ, utriusque, partem unam.
Syrupi aurantii corticis, partes quatuor.

Mannam prius in mortario contusam, calore leni, in syrupo solve : dein adde pulpas ; et perstante calore, ad crassitudinem idoneam vaporent.

CONFECTIO ROSÆ.

℞. Rosæ quantumvis.

In pulpam contunde, et sacchari, inter contundendum, pondus triplex adde.

CONFECTIO SCAMMONIÆ.

℞. Scammoniæ ;
Zingiberis, utriusque in pulverem redacti, unciam unam.
Caryophyllorum olei minima viginti.
Syrupi aurantii corticis quantum sit satis.

CONFECTION OF ORANGE PEEL.

Take of Fresh orange peel, one part.
  Sugar, three parts.

Bruise the peel to a pulp, gradually adding the sugar during the beating.

CONFECTION OF CASSIA.

Take of Purging cassia, four parts.
  Tamarind, the pulp ;
  Manna, of each, one part.
  Syrup of orange peel, four parts.

Having beat the manna in a mortar, dissolve it with a gentle heat in the syrup ; then add the pulps, and evaporate with regularly continued heat to a proper consistence.

CONFECTION OF ROSES.

COMMONLY CALLED CONSERVE OF ROSES.

Take of Roses, any quantity.

Beat them to a pulp ; and add, during the beating, three times their weight of sugar.

CONFECTION OF SCAMMONY.

Take of Scammony ;
  Ginger, of each in powder, one ounce.
  Oil of cloves, one fluid scruple.
  Syrup of orange peel, what is sufficient

14

In pulverem subtilissimum arida simul tere : dein inter syrupum gradatim addendum, iterum contere : tum caryophyllorum oleum adde ; et omnia commisce.

CONFECTIO SENNÆ.

R. Sennæ uncias octo.
    Coriandri uncias quatuor.
    Glycyrrhizæ contusæ uncias tres
    Ficuum libram unam.
    Prunorum libram unam.
    Tamarindi libram dimidiam.
    Sacchari libras duas cum semisse.

Sennam cum coriandro tere, et per cribrum separa pulveris misti uncias decem. Residuum cum ficibus et glycyrrhiza in quatuor octantibus aquæ decoque ad dimidiam ; dein exprime et cola. Liquorem colatum per vaporationem absume ad octantem circiter unam cum semisse. Postea adde saccharum ut fiat syrupus. Hunc syrupum adde gradatim pulpis ; et postremo immisce pulverem.

CUPRUM.

CUPRI AMMONIARETUM.

R. Cupri sulphatis partes duas.
    Ammoniæ carbonatis partes tres.

Diligenter subige in mortario vitreo, donec, finitâ omni effervescentiâ, placide coëant in massam violaceam ; quæ chartâ bibulâ obvoluta, primo super lapidem cretaceum, dein leni calore exsiccata, in vase vitreo bene obturato servetur.

Rub the dry articles together into a very fine powder; next rub them again while the syrup is gradually added; then add the oil of cloves, and mix the whole well together.

CONFECTION OF SENNA.

FORMERLY LENITIVE ELECTUARY.

Take of Senna, eight ounces.

        Coriander, three ounces.

        Liquorice, bruised, four ounces.

        Figs, one pound.

        Prunes, (the pulp,) one pound.

        Tamarind, half a pound.

        Sugar, two pounds and a half.

Pulverize the senna with the coriander, and sift out ten ounces of the mixed powder; boil the remainder with the figs and liquorice, in four pints of water, to one half; express and strain the liquor, which is then to be evaporated to about a pint and a half; dissolve the sugar in it, add this syrup by degrees to the pulps, and lastly mix in the sifted powder.

COPPER.

AMMONIARET OF COPPER.

Take of Sulphate of copper, two parts.

        Carbonate of ammonia, three parts.

Rub them diligently together in a glass mortar, until, after the effervescence has ceased, they unite into a violet coloured mass. This must be wrapped up in blotting paper, and first dried on a chalk stone, and afterwards by a gentle heat. The product must be kept in a glass phial well stopped.

CUPRI AMMONIARETI LIQUOR.

℞. Aquæ calcis octantem dimidium.
Ammoniæ muriatis scrupulos duos.
Cupri subacetatis præparati grana quatuor.

Misce et digere ad horas viginti quatuor ; deinde purum effunde liquorem.

CUPRI SUBACETAS PRÆPARATUM.

℞. Cupri subacetatis quantumvis.

In pulverem subige, et particulas minutas, ut in calcis carbonate præparando, separa.

CUPRI SULPHATIS LIQUOR.

℞. Cupri sulphatis grana tria.
Acidi sulphurici minima decem.
Aquæ distillatæ fluiduncias duas.

Misce, et agitando fiat solutio.

DECOCTA.

Decoctis utimur ad partes vegetabilium extrahendas quæ aquâ bullienti facilius solvantur, neque inter ebulliendum volatiles evanescant. Paranda sunt in vasis coopertis, calore non mutato. Inter parandum et utendum brevi tantum mora intersit.

SOLUTION OF AMMONIARET OF COPPER

Take of Lime water, half a pint.
Muriate of ammonia, two scruples.
Subacetate of copper, prepared, four grains.

Mix, and digest them for twenty-four hours, then pour off the pure liquor.

PREPARED SUBACETATE OF COPPER.

Take of Subacetate of copper, any quantity.

Grind it to powder, and separate the minute particles in the manner directed for the preparation of carbonate of lime.

SOLUTION OF SULPHATE OF COPPER.

Take of Sulphate of copper, three grains.
Sulphuric acid, ten minims.
Distilled water, two fluidounces.

Mix the articles, and effect a solution by shaking them.

DECOCTIONS.

Decoctions are used to extract those parts of vegetables which are most soluble in boiling water, and are not so volatile as to escape during the process.   Decoctions should be made in covered vessels, with a uniform heat, and prepared a short time before they are wanted for use.

DECOCTUM ARALIÆ NUDICAULIS.

℞. Araliæ nudicaulis contusæ uncias sex.
Aquæ octantes octo.

Digere per horas quatuor, tum decoque ad octantes quatuor, exprime et cola decoctum.

——◆——

DECOCTUM CINCHONÆ.

℞. Cinchonæ, in pulverem tritæ, unciam unam.
Aquæ octantem unum cum semisse.

Coque per horæ partem sextam in vase operto, et liquorem adhuc calentem cola.

——◆——

DECOCTUM COLOMBÆ COMPOSITUM.

℞. Colombæ contusæ ;
Quassiæ in scobem rasæ, utriusque drachmas duas.
Aurantii corticis drachmam unam.
Rhei in pulverem triti scrupulum unum.
Potassæ carbonatis drachmam dimidiam.
Aquæ fluiduncias viginti.

Coque ad octantem, et tincturæ lavandulæ adde fluidunciam dimidiam.

——◆——

DECOCTUM DULCAMARÆ.

℞. Dulcamaræ unciam unam.
Aquæ octantem cum semisse.

Decoque ad octantem, et cola.

DECOCTION OF FALSE SARSAPARILLA.

Take of False sarsaparilla, bruised, six ounces.
Water, eight pints.

Digest for four hours, and then boil down to four pints; press out and strain the decoction.

DECOCTION OF PERUVIAN BARK.

Take of Peruvian bark, in powder, one ounce.
Water, one pint and a half.

Boil for ten minutes, in a covered vessel, and strain the liquor while hot.

COMPOUND DECOCTION OF COLUMBO.

Take of Columbo, bruised ;
Quassia, rasped, of each, two drachms.
Orange peel, one drachm.
Rhubarb, in powder, one scruple.
Carbonate of potass, half a drachm.
Water, twenty fluidounces.

Boil to a pint, and add half a fluidounce of tincture of lavender.

DECOCTION OF BITTER SWEET.

Take of Bitter sweet, one ounce.
Water, one pint and a half.

Boil down to a pint, and strain.

DECOCTUM GUAIACI.

℞. Guaiaci ligni in scobem rasi uncias tres.
Uvarum uncias duas.
Sassafras concisi ;
Glycyrrhizæ contusæ, utriusque unciam unam.
Aquæ octantes decem.

Decoque leni igne lignum guaiaci et uvas in aqua ad octantes quinque, sub finem adjiciens radices ; dein cola sine expres-
sione.

DECOCTUM HORDEI.

℞. Hordei uncias duas.

Hordeum prius in aqua frigida lotum, coque per breve tempus
in aquæ circiter octante dimidio.   Aquâ hac abjectâ, hordeo octantes quinque aquæ ebullientis infunde.   Coque exin donec
aqua ad dimidium vaporet ; et postea cola.

DECOCTUM HORDEI COMPOSITUM.

℞. Decocti hordei octantes quatuor.
Uvarum, demptis acinis, uncias duas.
Ficuum discissarum uncias duas.
Glycyrrhizæ contusæ unciam dimidiam.

Liquorem ad dimidium decoque additis prius uvis, tum ficibus,
et, paulo ante finem coquendi, glycyrrhiza ; denique cola.

DECOCTION OF GUAIACUM.

FORMERLY DECOCTION OF THE WOODS.

Take of Guaiacum wood, rasped, three ounces.
    Raisins, two ounces.
    Sassafras, sliced ;
    Liquorice, bruised, of each, one ounce.
    Water, ten pints.

Boil the guaiacum and raisins in the water, over a gentle fire, down to five pints, adding the roots towards the end of the boiling ; then strain the liquor without expression.

DECOCTION OF BARLEY.

Take of Barley, two ounces.

Having first washed the barley in cold water, boil it for a short time in about half a pint of water ; throw away this water ; then pour upon the barley five pints of boiling water ; boil it next until half the quantity of the water be evaporated, and afterwards strain it.

COMPOUND DECOCTION OF BARLEY.

Take of Decoction of barley, four pints.
    Raisins, stoned, two ounces.
    Figs, sliced, two ounces.
    Liquorice, bruised, half an ounce.

Boil to the consumption of one half of the liquor ; first adding the raisins. then the figs, and, a short time before the process is finished, the liquorice ; lastly strain.

15

DECOCTUM LICHENIS.

R. Lichenis unciam unam.
Aquæ octantem cum semisse.

Decoque ad octantem, et exprimens cola.

DECOCTUM MEZEREI.

R. Mezerei drachmas duas.
Glycyrrhizæ contusæ unciam dimidiam.
Aquæ octantes tres.

Decoque leni igne ad octantes duos, et cola.

DECOCTUM SARSAPARILLÆ.

R. Sarsaparillæ concisæ uncias sex.
Aquæ congium unum.

Digere per duas horas, calore circiter gradus cxcv; dein ra-
dicem exime et contunde; contusam liquori redde, et decoque,
leni igne, ad quatuor octantes; tum exprime et cola.

DECOCTUM SARSAPARILLÆ COMPOSITUM.

R. Sarsaparillæ discissæ et contusæ unciam unam cum
semisse.
Guaiaci in scobem rasi;
Sassafras;
Glycyrrhizæ contusæ; singulorum drachmas duas.
Mezerei drachmam unam.
Aquæ bullientis octantes tres.

DECOCTION OF ICELAND MOSS.

Take of Iceland moss, one ounce.
Water, one pint and a half.

Boil down to a pint, and strain with compression.

———

DECOCTION OF MEZEREON.

Take of Mezereon, two drachms.
Liquorice, bruised, half an ounce.
Water, three pints.

Boil with a gentle heat to two pints, and strain.

———

DECOCTION OF SARSAPARILLA.

Take of Sarsaparilla, sliced, six ounces.
Water, one gallon.

Digest for two hours, with a heat of about 195; then take out the sarsaparilla, and bruise it; when bruised, put it back into the same liquor, boil down to four pints, then press out and strain the decoction.

———

COMPOUND DECOCTION OF SARSAPARILLA.

FORMERLY LISBON DIET DRINK.

Take of Sarsaparilla, sliced and bruised, one ounce and a half.
Guaiacum wood, rasped;
Sassafras;
Liquorice, bruised; of each, two drachms.
Mezereon, one drachm.
Boiling water, three pints.

Digere in aqua, calore leni. per horas sex, sarsaparillam, guaiacum et sassafras ; tum ad dimidium decoque, glycyrrhiza et mezereo, sub coquendi finem, additis ; et cola liquorem.

DECOCTUM SCILLÆ.

℞. Scillæ drachmas tres.
　　Juniperi uncias quatuor.
　　Senegæ uncias tres.
　　Aquæ octantes quatuor.

Coque ad consumendam liquoris dimidiam partem ; tum cola, et adde

　　　　Spiritus ætheris nitrosi fluiduncias quatuor.

DECOCTUM SENEGÆ.

℞. Senegæ unciam unam.
　　Aquæ octantes duos.

Decoque ad octantem, et cola.

DECOCTUM VERATRI.

℞. Veratri contriti unciam unam.
　　Aquæ octantes duas.
　　Alcoholis fluiduncias duas.

Decoque veratrum in aquâ ad octantem, et cola ; tum, postquam refrixerit, adjice alcohol.

Digest in the water, with a gentle heat, for six hours, the sarsaparilla, guaiacum, and sassafras ; then boil down to one half, adding towards the end of the boiling, the liquorice and mezereon ; and strain the liquor.

DECOCTION OF SQUILL.

Take of Squill, three drachms.
   Juniper, four ounces.
   Seneca snakeroot, three ounces.
   Water, four pints.

Boil to the consumption of one half the liquor ; then strain and add,
   Spirit of nitrous ether, four fluidounces.

DECOCTION OF SENECA SNAKEROOT.

Take of Seneca snakeroot, one ounce.
   Water, two pints.

Boil down to a pint, and strain.

DECOCTION OF WHITE HELLEBORE.

Take of White hellebore, powdered, one ounce.
   Water, two pints.
   Alcohol, two fluidounces.

Boil the hellebore in the water down to a pint. and strain the decoction ; then after it has cooled, add the alcohol.

EMPLASTRA.

Emplastra plerumque ex oleis et unguinosis parantur, oxidis seu pulveribus admixtis ad crassitudinem ut in frigore dura sint et digitis non adhæreant ; at in temperie corporis humani mollia et flexilia maneant, tamen ita glutinosa ut parti cui apponantur et materiæ in quam obducentur facile adhæreant. Ut emplastra facile obducentur, prius lento igne liquanda vel emollienda sunt.

EMPLASTRUM AMMONIACI.

R. Ammoniaci uncias quinque.
Aceti octantem dimidium.

Liqua ammoniacum in aceto, et exprime ; dein liquorem in vase ferreo, in balneo aquoso consume, assidue movens donec idonea fiat crassitudo.

EMPLASTRUM ASSAFŒTIDÆ.

R. Emplastri plumbi ;
Assafœtidæ utriusque partes duas.
Galbani ;
Ceræ flavæ utriusque partem unam.

Liquefac simul in balneo aquoso, et assidue move donec refrixerint.

PLASTERS.

Plasters are composed chiefly of oils and unctuous substances united with oxides or powders, into such consistence that the compound may remain firm in the cold without sticking to the fingers : that it may be soft and pliable in the heat of the human body ; yet so tenacious as readily to adhere both to the parts on which it is applied, and to the substance on which it is spread. Plasters require to be melted, or rather softened, by a gentle heat, to admit of their being spread.

AMMONIACUM PLASTER.

Take of Ammoniacum, five ounces.
   Vinegar, half a pint.

Dissolve the ammoniacum in the vinegar, and strain ; then evaporate the liquor in an iron vessel, by means of a water bath, constantly stirring it until it acquires a proper consistence.

ASSAFŒTIDA PLASTER.

Take of Lead plaster ;
   Assafœtida, each, two parts.
   Galbanum ;
   Yellow wax, each, one part.

Melt them together by means of a water bath, then stir them constantly until cool.

EMPLASTRUM FERRI.

℞. Emplastri plumbi partes viginti quatuor.
Resinæ pini partes sex.
Ceræ flavæ ;
Olivæ olei utriusque partes tres.
Ferri oxidi rubri partes octo.

Teratur ferri oxidum rubrum cum oleo, dein cæteris, in balneo aquoso liquefactis, adjiciatur.

EMPLASTRUM HYDRARGYRI.

℞. Olivæ olei ;
Resinæ pini utriusque partem unam.
Hydrargyri partes tres.
Emplastri plumbi partes sex.

Cum oleo et resina liquefactis simul et dein refrigeratis, teratur hydrargyrus donec evanescant globuli ; tum paulatim addatur emplastrum plumbi liquefactum et omnia accurate misceantur.

EMPLASTRUM PLUMBI.

℞. Plumbi oxidi semivitrei partem unam.
Olivæ olei partes duas.

Adjecta aqua coque, assidue agitans donec oleum et oxidum in emplastrum coëant.

PLASTER OF IRON.

STRENGTHENING PLASTER.

Take of Lead plaster, twenty-four parts.
        Pine resin, six parts.
        Yellow wax ;
        Olive oil, each, three parts.
        Red oxide of iron, eight parts.

Rub the red oxide of iron with the oil ; then add the other ingredients, previously melted in a water bath.

MERCURIAL PLASTER.

Take of Olive oil ;
        Pine resin, each, one part.
        Mercury, three parts.
        Lead plaster, six parts.

Rub the mercury with the oil and resin melted together, until the globules disappear ; then gradually add the lead plaster melted, and mix the whole intimately.

LEAD PLASTER.

Take of Semivitrified oxide of lead, one part.
        Olive oil, two parts.

Having added some water, boil them, constantly stirring until the oxide and oil unite into a plaster.

16

EMPLASTRUM PLUMBI SUBCARBONATIS COMPO SITUM.

    ℞. Plumbi subcarbonatis libram unam.
       Olivæ olei octantes duos.
       Ceræ flavæ uncias quatuor.
       Emplastri plumbi libram unam cum semisse.
       Iridis florentinæ in pulverem tritæ uncias novem.

Oleum et plumbum in balneo aquoso coque, assiduo agitans, donec unum corpus fiant : dein adjice ceram et emplastrum ; his liquefactis iridem insperge totum diligenter agitans.

EMPLASTRUM RESINOSUM.

    ℞. Emplastri plumbi partes quinque.
       Resinæ pini partem unam.

Liquefac simul in balneo aquoso, et assidue move donec refrixerint.

EMPLASTRUM RESINOSUM CANTHARIDUM.

    ℞. Cerati cantharidum partem unam.
       Picis abietis partes septem.

Liquefac simul in balneo aquoso, et assidue move donec refrixerint.

COMPOUND PLASTER OF SUBCARBONATE OF LEAD.

Take of Subcarbonate of lead, one pound.
 Olive oil, two pints
 Yellow wax, four ounces.
 Lead plaster, one pound and a half.
 Orris, in powder, nine ounces.

Boil the oil and lead together in a water bath, continually stirring, until they are thoroughly incorporated ; then add the wax and plaster ; and when these are melted, sprinkle in the powdered orris, carefully stirring the whole.

RESIN PLASTER.

ADHESIVE PLASTER.

Take of Lead plaster, five parts.
 Pine resin, one part.

Melt them together in a water bath, and stir them well until cold.

RESIN PLASTER WITH CANTHARIDES.

WARM PLASTER.

Take of Cerate of cantharides, one part.
 Burgundy pitch, seven parts.

Melt them together in a water bath, and stir them well until cold.

EXTRACTA.

Extracta ex vegetabilium succis et secretis, sive recentium, sive exsiccatorum parantur. Ad crassitudinem solidi, plus minusve mollis, rediguntur, recentia comprimendo et vaporando, arida autem in latice quovis solvendo, et postea solutum vaporando.

EXTRACTUM ACONITI.

℞. Aconiti recentis quantumvis.

In mortario lapideo contunde, et sacco cannabino inclusum, addito aquæ paululo, valide comprime, donec succum reddat. Hunc in vasis patulis, super balneo aquæ ferventis sodæ muriate prius saturatæ, illico ad mellis crassioris spissitudinem redige, sub finem spathula lignea agitans.

Postquam massa refrixerit reponatur in vasis fictilibus vitreatis, et alcohole madefiant.

Eodem modo parantur

EXTRACTUM BELLADONNÆ,

Ex belladonna recente.

EXTRACTUM CONII,

Ex conio recente.

EXTRACTS.*

Extracts are prepared from the juices and secretions of vegetables both in their recent and dried state. They are made in the form of a soft solid, from recent vegetables by expression and evaporation, and from dry ones by solution in a menstruum and subsequent evaporation.

EXTRACT OF ACONITE.

Take of Fresh aconite, any quantity.

Bruise it in a stone mortar, and having sprinkled on it a little water, press it strongly in a hempen bag till it yields its juice. This is to be evaporated immediately in flat vessels in a bath of boiling water saturated with muriate of soda, till it is brought to the consistence of thick honey. During the latter part of the process it should be stirred with a wooden spatula.

After the mass has become cold, it must be put up in glazed earthen vessels, and moistened with alcohol.

In like manner are prepared

EXTRACT OF DEADLY NIGHTSHADE,

From fresh deadly nightshade.

EXTRACT OF HEMLOCK,

From fresh hemlock.

* Under this head are included the Extracts and Inspissated Juices of former Pharmacopœias.

EXTRACTUM HYOSCYAMI,

Ex hyoscyamo recente.

EXTRACTUM STRAMONII,

Ex stramonio recente.

EXTRACTUM ANTHEMIDIS.

℞. Anthemidis siccatæ libram unam.
Aquæ congium unum.

Anthemidi affunde aquam, exin decoque ad octantes quatuor, et liquorem calentem exprimens cola. Decoctum illico per vaporationem redige ad mellis crassioris spissitudinem in balneo aquæ ferventis sodæ muriate saturatæ.

Postquam refrixerit extractum, in vasis fictilibus vitreatis, alcohole madefactis, reponatur.

Eodem modo parantur

EXTRACTUM GENTIANÆ,

Ex gentiana conscissa.

EXTRACTUM HÆMATOXYLI,

Ex hæmatoxylo in scobem raso.

EXTRACTUM HELLEBORI NIGRI.

Ex helleboro nigro conscisso.

EXTRACT OF HENBANE,

From fresh henbane.

EXTRACT OF THORN APPLE,

From fresh thorn apple.

EXTRACT OF CHAMOMILE.

Take of Dried chamomile, one pound.
Water, one gallon.

Pour the water upon the chamomile, boil down to four pints, and strain the liquor while hot, with compression. Evaporate the decoction immediately to the consistence of thick honey in a bath of boiling water, saturated with muriate of soda.

When the extract is cold, put it up in glazed earthen vessels, and moisten it with alcohol.

In like manner are prepared

EXTRACT OF GENTIAN,

From gentian cut in slices.

EXTRACT OF LOGWOOD,

From logwood, rasped.

EXTRACT OF BLACK HELLEBORE,

From black hellebore, sliced.

EXTRACTUM JUGLANDIS,

Ex juglande conscissa.

EXTRACTUM QUASSIÆ,

Ex quassia in scobem rasa.

EXTRACTUM CINCHONÆ.

℞. Cinchonæ in pulverem redactæ libram unam.
Alcoholis octantes quatuor.

Digere ad quatriduum et tincturam effunde.

Coque residuum in aquæ distillatæ octantibus quinque, ad partem horæ quartam ; et decoctum adhuc fervens per linteum cola. Denuo decoque in aquæ distillatæ octantibus alteris quinque, et cola ut antea ; dein, sedimento nullo ablato, liquorem vaporando, ad spissitudinem mellis tenuioris redige.

Alcohol a tinctura, donec hæc etiam similiter spissescat, distillando abstrahe ; dein liquores sic inspissatos misce ; et in aquæ ferventis balneo sodæ muriate saturatæ, ad crassitudinem idoneam vaporent.

EXTRACTUM COLOCYNTHIDIS COMPOSITUM.

℞. Colocynthidis conscissæ drachmas sex.
Aloes socotrinæ in pulverem redactæ unciam unam cum semisse.
Scammoniæ in pulverem redactæ unciam dimidiam.
Cardamomi in pulverem redacti drachmam unam.
Alcoholis diluti octantem unum.

Digere colocynthidem in alcohole per quatriduum calore leni. Solutioni colatæ aloen et scammoniam adde ; dein vaporet massa

EXTRACT OF BUTTERNUT,

From butternut sliced.

EXTRACT OF QUASSIA,

From quassia rasped.

EXTRACT OF PERUVIAN BARK.

Take of Peruvian bark, in powder, one pound.
Alcohol, four pints.

Digest for four days, and pour off the tincture.

Boil the residuum in five pints of distilled water, for fifteen minutes, and strain the decoction boiling hot, through linen. Repeat this decoction and filtration, with the same quantity of distilled water, and without any separation of sediment, reduce the liquor by evaporation to the consistence of thin honey.

Draw off the alcohol from the tincture by distillation, until this also becomes thick ; then mix the liquors thus inspissated, and evaporate them in a bath of boiling water, saturated with muriate of soda, to a proper consistence.

COMPOUND EXTRACT OF COLOCYNTH.

Take of Colocynth sliced, six drachms.
        Socotrine aloes powdered, one ounce and a half.
        Scammony powdered, half an ounce.
        Cardamom powdered, one drachm.
        Diluted alcohol, one pint.

Digest the colocynth in the diluted alcohol, for four days in a gentle heat ; strain the solution, and add to it the aloes and scam-

17

donec crassitudinis idoneæ fuerit ; et sub finem spissationis immisce cardamomum.

EXTRACTUM JALAPÆ.

R. Jalapæ contritæ libram unam.
Alcoholis octantes quatuor.
Aquæ octantes decem.

Macera jalapam in alcohole per quatriduum, et tincturam effunde. Residuum ex aquâ decoque ad octantes duos. Dein tincturam et decoctum separatim cola, et hoc consumatur, illa distillet, donec utrumque spissescat. Postremò commisceantur, et donec idonea fiat crassitudo, vaporando consumantur.

Servetur hoc extractum MOLLE, quod ad pilulas fingendas aptum sit, et DURUM, quòd in pulverem teri possit.

Hoc modo paratur

EXTRACTUM PODOPHYLLI.

EXTRACTUM SAMBUCI.

R. Sambuci baccas maturas, contunde, et succum exprime per saccum cannabinum, sive linteum ; succi hujus octantibus quinque sacchari libram unam adde ; et ad crassitudinem mellis crassioris vaporet.

mony; then evaporate the alcohol until the mass has acquired a proper consistence, and about the end of the inspissation, mix in the cardamom.

EXTRACT OF JALAP.

Take of Jalap powdered, one pound.
Alcohol, four pints.
Water, ten pints.

Macerate the jalap in the alcohol for four days, and pour off the tincture ; boil the remaining powder in the water until it be reduced to two pints ; then strain the tincture and decoction separately, and let the former be distilled, and the latter evaporated until each begins to grow thick. Lastly, mix the two together, and reduce to a proper consistence by evaporation.

Let this extract be kept in a SOFT state fit for forming pills, and in a HARD one so that it may be reduced to powder.

In the same way is prepared

EXTRACT OF MAY APPLE.

EXTRACT OF ELDER.

Take ripe elder berries, bruise them and press out the juice through a hempen or linen bag ; to five pints of this juice, add one pound of sugar, and evaporate to the consistence of thick honey.

FERRUM.

FERRI ACETAS.

℞. Ferri carbonatis præcipitati unciam dimidiam.
Aceti fluiduncias tres.

Digere per tres dies et cola.

FERRI CARBONAS PRÆCIPITATUS.

℞. Ferri sulphatis uncias octo.
Sodæ subcarbonatis uncias sex.
Aquæ bullientis congium unum.

Ferri sulphatem et sodæ subcarbonatem separatim liqua in aquæ octantibus quatuor ; tum liquores inter se misce, et sepone, ut pulvis subsidat ; deinde, effuso liquore supernatante, ferri carbonatem aquâ calidâ ablue, et chartâ bibulâ involutam leni calore exsicca.

FERRI CARBONAS PRÆPARATUS.

℞. Ferri limaturæ purificatæ, quantumvis.

Sæpius aquâ humectetur ut in rubiginem transeat, quæ in pollen teratur.

IRON.

—

ACETATE OF IRON.

Take of Precipitated carbonate of iron, half an ounce.
        Vinegar three fluidounces.

Digest for three days and strain.

———

PRECIPITATED CARBONATE OF IRON.

Take of Sulphate of iron, eight ounces.
        Subcarbonate of soda, six ounces.
        Boiling water, a gallon.

Dissolve the sulphate of iron, and subcarbonate of soda separately, each in four pints of water ; next mix the solutions together, and set the mixture by, that the precipitated powder
may subside ; then having poured off the supernatant liquor,
wash the carbonate of iron with hot water, and dry it upon bibulous paper in a gentle heat.

———

PREPARED CARBONATE OF IRON.

RUST OF IRON.

Take of Purified iron filings, any quantity.

Moisten them frequently with water, that they may be converted into rust, which is to be ground into an impalpable powder.

FERRI LIMATURA PURIFICATA.

℞. Ferri limaturæ quantumvis.

Imposito limaturæ cribro, admoveatur magnes, ut trans cribrum limatura sursum attrahatur.

AMMONIÆ ET FERRI MURIAS.

℞. Ferri oxidi rubri loti et exsiccati ;
Ammoniæ muriatis utriusque pondera paria.

Bene permista sublimentur.

FERRI OXIDUM RUBRUM.

℞. Ferri sulphatis quantumvis.

In vase fictili, non vitreato, calefiat igne modico, donec albescat et siccissimus fiat ; dein igne vehementi urgeatur, donec in materiam ruberrimam transierit.

FERRI PHOSPHAS.

℞. Ferri sulphatis uncias quatuor.
Aquæ octantes decem.

Solve, et requiescat solutum, donec fæces subsederint ; dein liquidum purum transfunde. In vase alio sodæ phosphatis uncias quatuor in aquæ octantibus tribus solve, et liquores misce. Pulverem cœruleum, qui præcipitatur, collige ; super colum pone ; dein aqua calente, donec hæc insipida evadat, ablue, et residuum calore modico sicca.

PURIFIED FILINGS OF IRON.

Take of Iron, in filings, any quantity.

Place a sieve over them, and apply a magnet, so that the filings may be attracted upwards through the sieve.

MURIATE OF AMMONIA AND IRON.

Take of Red oxide of iron, washed and dried ;
    Muriate of ammoniæ, of each, equal weights.

Mix them thoroughly, and sublime.

RED OXIDE OF IRON.

Take of Sulphate of iron, any quantity.

Expose it to the action of a moderate heat in an unglazed earthen vessel, until it becomes white and perfectly dry. Then expose it to an intense heat, until it is converted into a very red powder.

PHOSPHATE OF IRON.

Take of Sulphate of iron, four ounces.
    Water, ten pints.

Dissolve, and allow the solution to remain at rest until the impurities have subsided ; then decant the clear liquid. In a separate vessel dissolve four ounces of phosphate of soda, in three pints of water ; and mingle the two solutions. Collect the blue powder which is precipitated, place it on a filter, wash it with warm water, until the latter comes off tasteless, and dry the residue with a moderate heat.

LIQUOR FERRI ALKALINI.

℞. Ferri drachmas duas cum semisse.
Acidi nitrici fluiduncias duas.
Aquæ distillatæ fluiduncias sex.
Liquoris potassæ subcarbonatis fluiduncias sex.

Ferro superinfunde acidum et aquam inter se mista ; tum,
ubi bullulæ exire cessaverint, liquorem adhuc acidum effunde.
Hunc, paulatim et ex intervallis, liquori potassæ subcarbonatis
adjice, subinde agitans, donec, facto jam colore fusco-rubicundo,
bullulæ non amplius excitentur. Denique sepone per horas
sex, et liquorem effunde.

FERRI TARTRAS.

℞. Ferri carbonatis præcipitati unciam dimidiam.
Potassæ supertartratis in pulverem triti subtilissimum
unciam unam.
Aquæ distillatæ octantem unum.

Coque simul in vase vitreo super lentum ignem per horam
unam ; et liquorem per chartam cola. Liquor refrigeratus, et
iterum colatus, donec in superficie appareat pellicula, vaporet.
Inter frigescendum salina fiet massa, quæ in pulverem redigenda
est, et in vasis clausis servanda.

SOLUTION OF ALKALINE IRON.

Take of Iron, two drachms and a half.
Nitric acid, two fluidounces.
Distilled water, six fluidounces.
Solution of subcarbonate of potass, six fluidounces.

Having mixed the acid and water, pour them upon the iron, and when the effervescence has ceased, pour off the clear acid solution ; add this gradually, and at intervals, to the solution of subcarbonate of potass, occasionally shaking it, until it has assumed a deep brown red colour, and no further effervescence takes place. Lastly, set it by for six hours, and pour off the clear solution.

TARTRATE OF IRON.

Take of Precipitated carbonate of iron, half an ounce.
Supertartrate of potass, in very fine powder, one ounce.
Distilled water, one pint.

Boil them together in a glass vessel over a slow fire for an hour, and filter the liquor through paper. When cold, and filtered a second time, evaporate it until a pellicle appears on the surface. In cooling it will form a saline mass, which is to be powdered and kept in close vessels.

18

HYDRARGYRUM.

HYDRARGYRI OXIDUM CINEREUM.

℞. Hydrargyri submuriatis unciam unam.
Aquæ calcis congium unum.

Hydrargyri submuriatem in aquâ calcis coque, assiduè movens, ionec oxidum hydrargyri cinereum subsidat. Hoc aquâ
distillatâ lava, deinde exsicca.

HYDRARGYRI NITRICO-OXIDUM.

℞. Hydrargyri purificati libras tres.
Acidi nitrici libram unam cum semisse.
Aquæ distillatæ octantes duos.

Misce in vase vitreo ; et coque, donec liquetur hydrargyrum,
et, aquâ consumptâ, materia alba restet.   Hanc tere in pulverem, et in cucurbitam, scutellâ crassâ vitreâ superpositâ, injice.
Dein, capite adaptato, et vase in balneo arenæ posito, calorem
gradatim auctum accommoda, donec materies in squamas ruber-
rimas transierit.

HYDRARGYRI OXYMURIAS.

℞. Hydrargyri purificati libras duas.
Acidi sulphurici uncias triginta.
Sodæ muriatis exsiccati libras quatuor.

Hydrargyrum cum acido sulphurico in vase vitreo coque, donec hydrargyri sulphas exsiccatus fuerit ; hanc, ubi refrixerit,

MERCURY.

GREY OXIDE OF MERCURY.

Take of Submuriate of mercury, one ounce.
Lime water, one gallon.

Boil the submuriate of mercury in the lime water, constantly stirring, until a grey oxide is precipitated. Wash this with distilled water, and then dry it.

NITRĬC OXIDE OF MERCURY.
CALLED RED PRECIPITATE.

Take of Purified mercury, three pounds.
Nitric acid, one pound and a half.
Distilled water, two pints.

Mix in a glass vessel. Boil the mixture until the mercury is dissolved, and evaporate the solution with a gentle heat, to a dry white mass ; which, after being ground into powder, is to be put into a glass cucurbit, and to have a thick glass plate laid upon its surface. Then, having adapted a capital, and placed the vessel in a sand bath, apply a gradually increased heat, until the matter be converted into very red scales.

OXYMURIATE OF MERCURY.
CALLED CORROSIVE SUBLIMATE.

Take of Purified mercury, two pounds.
Sulphuric acid, thirty ounces.
Dried muriate of soda, four pounds.

Boil the mercury with the sulphuric acid in a glass vessel, until the sulphate of mercury is left dry. Rub this, when it is

cum sodæ muriate in mortario fictili contere ; tum ex cucurbitâ vitrea, calore sensim aucto, sublima.

LIQUOR HYDRARGYRI OXYMURIATIS.

℞. Hydrargyri oxymuriatis grana octo.
Aquæ distillatæ fluiduncias quindecim.
Alcoholis fluidunciam unum.

Hydrargyri oxymuriatem in aquâ liqua, eique adjice alcohol.

HYDRARGYRUM PURIFICATUM.

℞. Hydrargyri libras sex.
Ferri limaturæ libram unam.

Tere simul ; tum, igne subjecto, ex retortâ ferreâ distillet hydrargyrum.

HYDRARGYRI SUBMURIAS.

℞. Hydrargyri oxymuriatis libram unam.
Hydrargyri purificati uncias novem.

Tere simul, donec globuli non amplius conspiciantur ; tum sublima, deinde sublimatum exime, idque bis iterum et tere et sublima. Denique fiat pulvis subtilissimus, eodem modo quo calcis carbonatem præparari præceptum fuit.

cold, with the dried muriate of soda in an earthen ware mortar ; then sublime it in a glass cucurbit, increasing the heat gradually.

SOLUTION OF OXYMURIATE OF MERCURY.

Take of Oxymuriate of mercury, eight grains.
   Distilled water, fifteen fluidounces.
   Alcohol, one fluidounce.

Dissolve the oxymuriate of mercury in the water, and add the alcohol.

PURIFIED MERCURY.

Take of Mercury, six pounds.
   Iron, reduced to filings, one pound.

Rub them together and distil the mercury in an iron retort.

SUBMURIATE OF MERCURY.

CALLED CALOMEL.

Take of Oxymuriate of mercury, one pound.
   Purified mercury, nine ounces.

Rub them together till the metallic globules disappear ; then sublime, take out the sublimed mass, and reduce it to powder, and sublime it in the same manner twice more successively. Lastly, bring it into the state of a very fine powder, by the same process which has been directed for the preparation of carbonate of lime.

HYDRARGYRI SUBMURIAS AMMONIATUS.

R. Hydrargyri oxymuriatis libram dimidiam.
Ammoniæ muriatis uncias quatuor.
Liquoris potassæ subcarbonatis octantem dimidium.
Aquæ distillatæ octantes quatuor.

Primò ammoniæ muriatem, dein hydrargyri oxymuriatem, in aquâ distillatâ, liqua, et his adjice liquorem potassæ subcarbonatis. Pulverem demissum lava, donec saporis expers fuerit ; et dein exsicca.

———

HYDRARGYRI SUBSULPHAS FLAVUS.

R. Hydrargyri purificati uncias quatuor.
Acidi sulphurici uncias sex.

Indantur cucurbitæ vitreæ et coquantur ex arena ad siccitatem. Materia alba, in fundo relicta, trita, conjiciatur in aquam bullientem. Inde nascetur illico pulvis flavus, quem aquâ calidâ sæpius lavare oportet.

———

HYDRARGYRI SULPHURETUM NIGRUM.

R. Hydrargyri purificati ;
Sulphuris utriusque pondera æqualia.

Terantur simul in mortario vitreo, pistillo vitreo, donec globuli hydrargyri visum penitus effugerint.

AMMONIATED SUBMURIATE OF MERCURY.

FORMERLY WHITE PRECIPITATE.

Take of Oxymuriate of mercury, half a pound.
  Muriate of ammonia, four ounces.
  Solution of subcarbonate of potass, half a pint.
  Distilled water, four pints.

First dissolve the muriate of ammonia, then the oxymuriate of mercury, in the distilled water, and add thereto the subcarbonate of potass in solution. Wash the precipitated powder until it becomes tasteless ; then dry it.

YELLOW SUBSULPHATE OF MERCURY.

FORMERLY TURPETH MINERAL.

Take of Purified mercury, four ounces.
  Sulphuric acid, six ounces.

Put them into a glass cucurbit, and boil them in a sand bath to dryness. Throw into boiling water the white matter, which is left in the bottom, after having reduced it to powder. A yellow powder will immediately be produced, which must be frequently washed with warm water.

BLACK SULPHURET OF MERCURY.

FORMERLY ÆTHIOP'S MINERAL.

Take of Purified mercury ;
  Sulphur, of each, equal weights.

Grind them together in a glass mortar, with a glass pestle, till the globules entirely disappear.

HYDRARGYRI SULPHURETUM RUBRUM.

℞. Hydrargyri purificati uncias quadraginta.
Sulphuris uncias octo.

Sulphuri ad ignem liquefacto hydrargyrum admisce, et, quam primùm intumescat massa, vas ab igne remove, et arctius tege, ne fiat inflammatio ; deinde in pulverem tere, et sublima.

INFUSA.

Infusa esse volumus, in quibus vegetabilium partes aquâ vel calidâ vel frigidâ, sine bulliendo solvuntur. Si aquâ calidâ utendum est, tum vase cooperto in loco calido per tempus præscriptum macerare oportet.

Breve tantum tempus inter parandum et utendum interesse liceat.

INFUSUM ANGUSTURÆ.

℞. Angusturæ contusæ drachmas duas.
Aquæ bullientis octantem dimidium.

Macera per horas duas in vase levitèr clauso, et cola.

INFUSUM ANTHEMIDIS.

℞. Anthemidis drachmas duas.
Aquæ frigidæ octantem dimidium.

Macera per horas octo, in vase levitèr clauso, et cola.

RED SULPHURET OF MERCURY.
FORMERLY CINNABAR.

Take of Purified mercury, forty ounces.
Sulphur, eight ounces.

Having melted the sulphur over the fire, mix in the mercury, and as soon as the mass begins to swell, remove the vessel from the fire, and cover it with considerable force, to prevent combustion ; then rub the mass into powder, and sublime.

INFUSIONS.

Infusions are solutions made from vegetables either with hot or cold water, without boiling. If hot water is employed the infusion must be carried on in covered vessels, and in a warm place.

Infusions should be prepared only a short time before they are used.

INFUSION OF ANGUSTURA.

Take of Angustura, bruised, two drachms.
Boiling water, half a pint.

Infuse for two hours in a covered vessel, and strain.

INFUSION OF CHAMOMILE.

Take of Chamomile, two drachms.
Cold water, half a pint.

Macerate for eight hours in a covered vessel, and strain.

19

INFUSUM ARMORACIÆ.

℞. Armoraciæ concisæ ;
  Sinapis contusæ, utriusque unciam unam.
  Aquæ bullientis octantem unum.

Macera per horas duas, in vase levitèr clauso, et cola.

INFUSUM CASCARILLÆ.

℞. Cascarillæ contusæ unciam dimidiam.
  Aquæ bullientis octantem dimidium.

Macera per horas duas, in vase levitèr clauso, et cola.

INFUSUM CINCHONÆ.

℞. Cinchonæ contusæ unciam dimidiam.
  Aquæ bullientis octantem dimidium.

Macera per horas duas, in vase levitèr clauso, et cola.

INFUSUM CINCHONÆ CUM AQUA CALCIS.

℞. Cinchonæ in pulverem tritæ unciam unam.
  Aquæ calcis octantem unum.

Aquam calcis paulatim adde, et simul contere ad partem horæ quartam. Requiescat ad horam unam infusum, deinde coletur.

INFUSION OF HORSERADISH.

Take of Horseradish, sliced ;
    Mustard, bruised, of each, one ounce.
    Boiling water, one pint.

Infuse for two hours in a covered vessel, and strain.

INFUSION OF CASCARILLA.

Take of Cascarilla, bruised, half an ounce.
    Boiling water, half a pint.

Infuse for two hours in a covered vessel, and strain.

INFUSION OF PERUVIAN BARK.

Take of Peruvian bark, bruised, half an ounce.
    Boiling water, half a pint.

Infuse for two hours in a covered vessel, and strain.

INFUSION OF PERUVIAN BARK WITH LIME WATER.

Take of Peruvian bark, in powder, one ounce.
    Lime water, one pint.

Add the lime water gradually, and rub them well together for fifteen minutes. Let the infusion stand for one hour, then filter.

INFUSUM CINCHONÆ CUM MAGNESIA.

℞. Cinchonæ in pulverem tritæ unciam unam.
Magnesiæ drachmam unam.
Aquæ frigidæ octantem unum.

Aquam adde paulatim, et simul contere per horæ partem quartam. Requiescat ad horam unam infusum, deinde coletur.

—●—

INFUSUM CINCHONÆ CUM SUCCO LIMONUM.

℞. Cinchonæ in pulverem tritæ unciam unam.
Succi limonum fluiduncias duas.
Tincturæ camphoræ opiatæ fluidrachmas tres,
Aquæ frigidæ octantem unum.

Macera per horas duodecim in vase operto, et cola.

—●—

INFUSUM COLOMBÆ.

℞. Colombæ concisæ drachmam unam.
Aquæ bullientis octantem dimidium.

Macera per horas duas in vase levitèr clauso, et cola.

—●—

INFUSUM DIGITALIS.

℞. Digitalis siccatæ drachmam unam.
Aquæ bullientis octantem dimidium.
Tincturæ cinnamomi fluidunciam unam.

Digitalem per horas quatuor in vase cooperto macera ; cola, et cinnamomi tincturam adde.

INFUSION OF PERUVIAN BARK WITH MAGNESIA.

Take of Peruvian bark, in powder, one ounce.
 Magnesia, one drachm.
 Cold water, one pint.

Add the water gradually, and rub them well together for fifteen minutes. Let the infusion stand for one hour, then filter.

INFUSION OF PERUVIAN BARK WITH LEMON JUICE.

Take of Peruvian bark, in powder, one ounce.
 Juice of lemons, two fluidounces.
 Opiated tincture of camphor, three fluidrachms.
 Cold water, one pint.

Macerate for twelve hours in a covered vessel, and strain.

INFUSION OF COLUMBO.

Take of Columbo, sliced, one drachm.
 Boiling water, half a pint.

Infuse for two hours in a covered vessel, and strain.

INFUSION OF FOXGLOVE.

Take of Foxglove, dried, one drachm.
 Boiling water, half a pint.
 Tincture of cinnamon, one fluidounce.

Infuse the foxglove for four hours in a covered vessel, strain, and add the tincture of cinnamon.

INFUSUM EUPATORII.

℞. Eupatorii perfoliati unciam unam.
Aquæ bullientis octantem unum.

Macera per horas duas in vase levitèr clauso, et cola.

INFUSUM GENTIANÆ COMPOSITUM.

℞. Gentianæ concisæ unciam dimidiam.
Aurantii corticis contusi drachmam unam.
Coriandri contusi drachmam dimidiam.
Alcoholis diluti fluiduncias quatuor.
Aquæ frigidæ octantem unum.

Alcohol dilutum primo cæteris infunde ; et post horas tres, aquam adde : deinde per horas duodecim macera, et cola.

INFUSUM LINI.

℞. Lini seminùm contritorum unciam unam.
Glycyrrhizæ contusæ unciam dimidiam.
Aquæ bullientis octantes duos.

Macera per horas quatuor in vase levitèr clauso, et cola.

INFUSUM QUASSIÆ.

℞. Quassiæ rasæ drachmam unam.
Aquæ frigidæ octantem dimidium.

Macera per horas duodecim, et cola.

INFUSION OF THOROUGHWORT.

Take of Thoroughwort, one ounce.
Boiling water, one pint.

Infuse for two hours in a covered vessel, and strain.

COMPOUND INFUSION OF GENTIAN.

Take of Gentian, sliced, half an ounce.
Orange peel, bruised, one drachm.
Coriander, bruised, half a drachm.
Diluted alcohol, four fluidounces.
Cold water, one pint.

First, pour the diluted alcohol on the articles, and, three hours after add the water ; then macerate for twelve hours, and strain.

INFUSION OF FLAXSEED.

Take of Flaxseed, in meal, one ounce.
Liquorice, bruised, half an ounce.
Boiling water, two pints.

Infuse for four hours in a covered vessel, and strain.

INFUSION OF QUASSIA.

Take of Quassia, rasped, one drachm.
Cold water, half a pint.

Macerate for twelve hours, and strain.

INFUSUM QUASSIÆ CUM SULPHATE ZINCI.

℞. Quassiæ rasæ drachmam unam.
Zinci sulphatis grana octo.
Aquæ frigidæ octantem dimidium.

Macera per horas duodecim, et cola.

INFUSUM ROSÆ COMPOSITUM.

℞. Rosæ siccatæ unciam dimidiam.
Aquæ bullientis octantes duos cum semisse.
Acidi sulphurici diluti fluidrachmas tres.
Sacchari unciam unam cum semisse.

Aquam rosæ superinfunde in vase vitreo ; dein acidum immisce, et macera per horam dimidiam.   Denique liquorem cola,
et saccharum adjice.

INFUSUM SENNÆ COMPOSITUM.

℞. Sennæ unciam unam cum semisse.
Potassæ supertartratis drachmas duas,
Zingiberis drachmam unam.
Aquæ bullientis octantem unum.

Macera per horam unam in vase levitèr clauso, et cola.

INFUSUM SENNÆ ET TAMARINDI.

℞. Sennæ drachmam unam.
Tamarindi unciam unam.
Coriandri contusi drachmam dimidiam.
Sacchari unciam dimidiam.
Aquæ bullientis octantem dimidium.

INFUSION OF QUASSIA WITH SULPHATE OF ZINC.

Take of Quassia, rasped, one drachm.
    Sulphate of zinc, eight grains.
    Cold water, half a pint.

Macerate for twelve hours, and strain.

COMPOUND INFUSION OF ROSES.

Take of Roses, dried, half an ounce.
    Boiling water, two pints and a half.
    Diluted sulphuric acid, three fluidrachms.
    Sugar, one ounce and a half.

Pour the water upon the roses in a glass vessel ; then mix in the acid, and infuse for half an hour.   Lastly strain the infusion, and add the sugar to it.

COMPOUND INFUSION OF SENNA.

Take of Sennà, one ounce and a half.
    Supertartrate of potass, two drachms.
    Ginger, one drachm.
    Boiling water, one pint.

Infuse for an hour in a covered vessel, and strain.

INFUSION OF SENNA AND TAMARIND.

Take of Senna, one drachm.
    Tamarind, one ounce.
    Coriander, bruised, half a drachm.
    Sugar, half an ounce.
    Boiling water, half a pint.

20

Macera per horas quatuor, nonnunquam agitans, in vase clauso fictili, non plumbo vitreato, et cola.

INFUSUM SERPENTARIÆ.

℞. Serpentariæ unciam dimidiam.
    Aquæ bullientis octantem dimidium.

Macera per horas duas in vase leviter clauso, et cola.

INFUSUM SPIGELIÆ.

℞. Spigeliæ drachmas duas.
    Aquæ bullientis octantem dimidium.

Macera per horas quatuor in vase levitèr clauso, et cola.

INFUSUM TABACI.

℞. Tabaci drachmam unam.
    Aquæ bullientis octantem unum.

Macera per horam unam in vase levitèr clauso, et cola.

INFUSUM ULMI.

℞. Ulmi concisæ unciam unam.
    Aquæ bullientis octantem unum.

Macera per horas duodecim in vase clauso, sæpe agitans, et cola.

Infuse for four hours, with occasional agitation, in a close earthen vessel not glazed with lead, and strain.

INFUSION OF VIRGINIA SNAKEROOT.

Take of Virginia snakeroot, half an ounce.
Boiling water, half a pint.

Infuse for two hours in a covered vessel, and strain.

INFUSION OF CAROLINA PINK.

Take of Carolina pink, two drachms.
Boiling water, half a pint.

Infuse for four hours in a covered vessel, and strain.

INFUSION OF TOBACCO.

Take of Tobacco, one drachm.
Boiling water, one pint.

Infuse for one hour in a covered vessel, and strain.

INFUSION OF SLIPPERY ELM.

Take of Slippery elm, sliced, one ounce.
Boiling water, one pint.

Infuse for twelve hours in a covered vessel, near the fire with frequent agitation, and strain.

INFUSUM VALERIANÆ.

℞. Valerianæ drachmas duas.
    Aquæ bullientis octantem dimidium.

Macera per horam unam in vase leviter clauso, et cola.

LINIMENTA.

Linimenta plerumque ex oleis parantur, et, ut cuti facile il-
linantur, penitus fluida esse debent.

LINIMENTUM AMMONIÆ.

℞. Aquæ ammoniæ ;
    Olivæ olei utriusque partem æquam.

Misce.

LINIMENTUM AMMONIÆ ET ANTIMONII TAR-
TARIZATI.

℞. Linimenti ammoniæ fluidunciam unam.
    Ammonii tartarizati drachmam unam.

Misce.

INFUSION OF VALERIAN.

Take of Valerian, two drachms.
Boiling water, half a pint.

Infuse for an hour in a covered vessel, and strain.

LINIMENTS.

Liniments are generally prepared from oily substances, and are in a fluid state, as they are to be rubbed on the body.

LINIMENT OF AMMONIA.

Take of Water of ammonia ;
Olive oil, equal parts.

Mix.

LINIMENT OF AMMONIA WITH TARTARIZED ANTIMONY.

Take of Liniment of ammonia, one fluidounce.
Tartarized antimony, one drachm.

Mix.

LINIMENTUM AQUÆ CALCIS.

℞. Lini olei ;
Aquæ calcis, utriusque partem æquam.

Misce.

LINIMENTUM CAMPHORATUM.

℞. Camphoræ per alcohol in pulverem redactæ unciam
dimidiam.
Olivæ olei fluiduncias quatuor.

Misce.

LINIMENTUM CANTHARIDUM.

℞. Cantharidum in pulverem tritarum unciam unam.
Terebinthinæ olei fluiduncias octo.

Fervescant per horas tres, dein colantur.

LINIMENTUM SAPONIS CAMPHORATUM.

℞. Saponis albi rasi uncias duodecim.
Camphoræ uncias duas.
Olei volatilis rorismarini fluidrachmas duas.
Alcoholis congium unum.

Digere saponem in alcohole per triduum ; dein liquori colato,
adde camphoram et oleum, diligenter agitans.

LINIMENT OF LIME WATER.

Take of Flaxseed oil ;
    Lime water, each equal parts.

Mix.

CAMPHORATED LINIMENT.

Take of Camphor reduced to a powder by means of alcohol,
    half an ounce.
    Olive oil, four fluidounces.

Mix.

LINIMENT OF CANTHARIDES.

Take of Cantharides, in powder, one ounce.
    Oil of turpentine, eight fluidounces.

Simmer for three hours, then set by to cool, and filter.

CAMPHORATED SOAP LINIMENT.
OPODELDOC.

Take of Castile soap uncoloured, in shavings, twelve ounces.
    Camphor, two ounces.
    Volatile oil of rosemary, two fluidrachms.
    Alcohol, one gallon.

Digest the soap in the alcohol for three days, then filter, and
add the camphor and oil, mixing them intimately

LINIMENTUM SAPONIS ET OPII

Eodem modo, ut supra, paratur, adjecta opii uncia una, quæ cum sapone et alcohole digerenda est.

LINIMENTUM TABACI.

R. Tabaci concisi unciam unam.
Adipis libram unam.

Adipi incoque tabacum super ignem lenem donec friabile fiat ; tum per linteum exprime.

LINIMENTUM TEREBINTHINÆ COMPOSITUM.

R. Cerati resinosi libram unam.
Terebinthinæ olei octantem dimidium.

Liquefacto cerato adjice oleum terbinthinæ, et misce.

MAGNESIA.

MAGNESIA.

R. Magnesiæ carbonatis quantumvis.

Crucibulo inditus, igne rubescat per horas duas ; dein in vasis vitreis bene obturatis servetur.

LINIMENT OF SOAP AND OPIUM

Is prepared in the same way, by adding an ounce of opium, and digesting it with the soap and alcohol.

TOBACCO LINIMENT.

Take of Tobacco, cut fine, one ounce.
Hog's lard, one pound.

Simmer the tobacco in the lard over a gentle fire until it becomes crisp, and strain.

COMPOUND LINIMENT OF TURPENTINE.

Take of Resinous cerate, one pound.
Oil of turpentine, half a pint

Melt the cerate, and add the oil of turpentine.

MAGNESIA.

MAGNESIA.

Take of Carbonate of magnesia, any quantity.

Heat it to redness in a crucible, and keep it in this state for two hours. Then inclose it in well stopped glass bottles.

MELLITA.

MEL DESPUMATUM.

℞. Mellis quantumvis.

In balneo aquoso liqua ; tum spumam aufer.

MEL SCILLÆ ACETATUM.

℞. Mellis despumati libras tres.
Aceti scillæ octantes duos.

Decoque in vase vitreo ad crassitudinem idoneam aquæ balneo, sodæ muriate saturato.

MEL SCILLÆ COMPOSITUM.

℞. Scillæ siccatæ et contusæ ;
Senegæ contusæ, utriusque uncias quatuor.
Aquæ octantes quatuor.

Coque igne leni ad consumendam aquam dimidiam ; cola, et adde mellis despumati, libras duas   deinde coque ad octantes tres, et in uncia quaque hujus liquoris solve antimonii tartarizati granum unum.

PREPARED HONEYS.

CLARIFIED HONEY.

Take of Honey, any quantity.

Melt it by means of a water bath, then take off the scum.

ACETATED HONEY OF SQUILL.

CALLED OXYMEL OF SQUILL.

Take of Clarified honey, three pounds.
Vinegar of squill, two pints.

Boil them down, in a glass vessel, to a proper consistence, on a water bath, saturated with muriate of soda.

COMPOUND HONEY OF SQUILL.

Take of Squill, dried and bruised ;
Seneca snakeroot, bruised, of each four ounces.
Water, four pints.

Boil over a gentle fire, till the water is half consumed ; strain, and add, of clarified honey, two pounds ; boil to three pints, and dissolve in every ounce of this liquor one grain of tartarized antimony.

MISTURÆ.

MISTURA AMMONIACI.

Ammoniaci drachmas duas.
Aquæ octantom dimidium.

Tere ammoniacum cum aquâ paulatim instillatâ, donec quam optime misceantur.

MISTURA AMYGDALÆ.

R. Amygdalarum unciam unam.
Sacchari purificati unciam dimidiam.
Aquæ octantes duos cum semisse.

Amygdalas decorticatas in mortario lapideo diligenter contunde, aquam simul paulatim affundens ; dein cola.

MISTURA AMMONIACI ET ANTIMONII.

R. Misturæ ammoniaci fluiduncias quatuor.
Vini antimonii tartarizati fluidrachmas quatuor.
Syrupi Tolutani fluidunciam unam.
Tincturæ camphoræ opiatæ fluidrachmas quatuor.
Misce.

MISTURA CALCIS CARBONATIS.

R. Calcis carbonatis præparati unciam unam cum semisse.
Sacchari unciam unam.
Acaciæ gummi in pulverem triti unciam dimidiam.
Olei cinnamomi minima decem.
Aquæ fluiduncias viginti.

MIXTURES.

AMMONIACUM MIXTURE.

Take of Ammoniacum, two drachms.
 Water, half a pint.

Rub the ammoniacum with the water gradually poured upon it, until they are perfectly mixed.

ALMOND MIXTURE.

Take of Almonds, an ounce.
 Refined sugar, half an ounce.
 Water, two pints and a half.

Beat the almonds, when blanched, thoroughly in a stone mortar, gradually pouring on them the water ; then strain.

MIXTURE OF AMMONIACUM AND ANTIMONY.
WHITE MIXTURE.

Take of Ammoniacum mixture, four fluidounces.
 Wine of antimony, four fluidrachms.
 Syrup of Tolu, one fluidounce.
 Opiated tincture of camphor, four fluidrachms.
Mix.

MIXTURE OF CARBONATE OF LIME.

Take of Prepared carbonate of lime, one ounce and a half.
 Sugar, one ounce.
 Acacia gum, in powder, half an ounce.
 Oil of cinnamon, ten minims.
 Water, twenty fluidounces.

Acaciæ gummi subige cum aquæ flidunciis quatuor. Deinde tere oleum cum saccharo et omnia misce.

MISTURA CAMPHORÆ.

℞. Camphoræ drachmam dimidiam.
    Alcoholis minima decem.
    Sacchari unciam dimidiam.
    Aquæ octantem unum.

Camphoram primum cum alcohole tere, deinde cum aqua paulatim instillatâ, et cola.

MISTURA FERRI COMPOSITA.

℞. Myrrhæ in pulverem tritæ drachmam unam.
    Potassæ subcarbonatis grana viginti quinque.
    Aquæ rosæ octantem dimidium.
    Ferri sulphatis in pulverem triti scrupulum unum.
    Spiritus lavandulæ flidunciam dimidiam.
    Sacchari drachmam unam.

Myrrham cum potassæ subcarbonate et saccharo simul tere, hisque dum conteruntur, primum aquam rosæ et spiritum lavandulæ, postremo ferri sulphatem adjice. Misturam statim in vas vitreum immitte, idque obtura.

MISTURA MAGNESIÆ.

℞. Magnesiæ drachmam unam.
    Aquæ ammoniæ carbonatis fluidrachmam unam.
    Aquæ cinnamomi fluidrachmas tres.
    Aquæ distillatæ fliduncias quinque cum semisse.

Misce.

Rub down the gum with four ounces of water. Then rub the oil with the sugar, and afterwards mix the whole together.

CAMPHOR MIXTURE.

Take of Camphor, half a drachm.
  Alcohol, ten minims.
  Sugar, half an ounce.
  Water, one pint.

First rub the camphor with the alcohol, then with the water gradually added, and strain the liquor.

COMPOUND MIXTURE OF IRON.
CALLED MYRRH MIXTURE.

Take of Myrrh, in powder, one drachm.
  Subcarbonate of potass, twenty-five grains.
  Rose water, half a pint.
  Sulphate of iron, in powder, one scruple.
  Spirit of lavender, half a fluidounce.
  Sugar, one drachm.

Rub together the myrrh, the subcarbonate of potass and su-gar, and during the trituration, add gradually, first the rose wa-ter and spirit of lavender, and lastly the sulphate of iron. Pour the mixture immediately into a suitable glass bottle, and stop it close.

MAGNESIA MIXTURE.

Take of Magnesia, one drachm.
  Water of carbonate of ammonia, one fluidrachm.
  Cinnamon water, three fluidrachms.
  Distilled water five fluidounces and a half.

Mix.

MISTURA MOSCHI.

R. Moschi ;
     Acaciæ gummi in pulverem triti.
     Sacchari purificati, singulorum drachmam unam.
     Aquæ rosæ fluiduncias sex.

Tere moschum cum saccharo, deinde cum gummi, instillatâ
paulatim aquâ rosæ.

MISTURA ZINCI SULPHATIS.

R. Zinci sulphatis drachmas duas.
     Spiritus lavandulæ fluidrachmas duas.
     Aquæ fluiduncias sex.

Misce.

OLEA DISTILLATA.

In oleis volatilibus parandis introducatur materia, ex quâ
oleum derivandum sit, in retortam, seu vas quodque ad distillan-
dum idoneum ; et aquæ ad materiam tegendam satis infunde-
tur : deinde oleum in vas amplum refrigeratorium distillet.

Oleum cum aqua transvectum postea separandum est, prout
aquâ levius, summâ supernatet seu gravius imum petat.

Hoc modo paranda sunt

OLEUM ANISI,

Ab aniso.

OLEUM CHENOPODII,

A chenopodio.

MUSK MIXTURE.

Take of Musk ;
  Acacia gum, in powder;
  Refined sugar, each, one drachm.
  Rose water, six fluidounces.

Rub the musk first with the sugar, then with the gum, and add the rose water by degrees.

SULPHATE OF ZINC MIXTURE.

Take of Sulphate of zinc, two drachms.
  Spirit of lavender, two fluidrachms.
  Water, six fluidounces.
Mix.

DISTILLED OILS.

In preparing such oils as are volatile, we introduce the substance from which the oil is to be obtained, into a retort or common still, and pour on as much water as will cover it ; then distil into a large refrigeratory.

The oil comes over with the water, and is afterwards to be separated from it, according as it may be lighter than the water, and swim upon its surface, or heavier, and sink to the bottom.

According to the above method are prepared
OIL OF ANISE,
From anise.

OIL OF WORMSEED
From wormseed.

22

⊖LEUM CUNILÆ,

A cunila.

———

OLEUM FŒNICULI,

A fœniculo.

———

OLEUM GAULTHERIÆ,

A gaultheria.

———

OLEUM JUNIPERI,

A junipero.

———

OLEUM LAVANDULÆ,

A lavandula.

———

OLEUM MENTHÆ PIPERITÆ,

A mentha piperita.

———

OLEUM MENTHÆ VIRIDIS,

A mentha viridi.

———

OLEUM MONARDÆ,

A monarda.

———

OLEUM ORIGANI,

Ab origano.

———

OLEUM PIMENTÆ,

A pimenta.

———

OLEUM RORISMARINI,

A roremarino.

OIL OF PENNYROYAL,

From pennyroyal.

OIL OF FENNEL,

From fennel.

OIL OF PARTRIDGE BERRY,

From partridge berry.

OIL OF JUNIPER,

From juniper.

OIL OF LAVENDER,

From lavender.

OIL OF PEPPERMINT,

From peppermint.

OIL OF SPEARMINT,

From spearmint.

OIL OF MONARDA,

From monarda.

OIL OF ORIGANUM,

From marjoram.

OIL OF PIMENTO,

From pimento.

OIL OF ROSEMARY,

From rosemary.

OLEUM SASSAFRAS,

A sassafras.

OLEUM SUCCINI.

℞. Succini quantumvis, in pulverem redacti subtilem
cum arenæ puræ pari pondere.

In retortam vitream immitte et ex iis distillent in arenæ balneo, calore gradatim aucto, liquor acidus, oleum, et sal oleo-
sum.

Deinde oleum cum aquâ quantitatem suam sexies superante,
iterum distillet, donec in excipulum aquæ bis triens transierit.
Oleum ab aqua separa, et in vasis bene obturatis serva.

OLEUM SUCCINI OXIDATUM.

℞. Olei succini fluidrachmam unam.
Acidi nitrici fluidrachmas tres cum semisse.

Oleum succini in vas vitreum mitte, et acidum guttatim instilla, misturam eodem tempore spatha vitrea movens. Per horas
triginta sex requiescat, dein ab acido fluido resinosum supernatans separa ; et primo in aqua frigida, et denique in aqua
calida ablue, donec sapor acidulus evanuerit.

OIL OF SASSAFRAS,

From sassafras.

OIL OF AMBER.

Take of Amber, any quantity, reduced to a fine powder, with an equal weight of clean sand.

Put them into a glass retort, and distil from them in a sand bath, with a gradually increased heat, an acid liquor, oil, and salt impregnated with oil.

Re-distil the oil, with six times its quantity of water, till two thirds of the water have passed into the receiver; then separate the volatile oil from the water, and preserve it in well stopped phials.

OXIDATED OIL OF AMBER.

Take of Oil of amber, one fluidrachm.
Nitric acid, three and a half fluidrachms.

Put the oil of amber into a glass vessel, and gradually drop the acid into it, at the same time stirring the mixture with a glass rod. Let it stand for thirty-six hours, then separate the supernatant resinous matter from the acid fluid beneath, and wash it repeatedly, first with cold, and lastly with hot water, till the acid taste disappears.

PILULÆ.

PILULÆ ALOETICÆ.

℞. Aloës socotrinæ in pulverem tritæ ;
 Saponis, utriusque partem æqualem.

Subige cum aquâ, ut fiat massa ad pilulas formandas idonea.

PILULÆ ALOES ET COLOCYNTHIDIS.

℞. Aloës socotrinæ ;
 Scammoniæ utriusque uncias duas.
 Potassæ sulphatis drachmas duas.
 Colocynthidis unciam unam.
 Caryophyllorum olei fluidrachmas duas.

Aloën et scammoniam cum potassæ sulphate in pulverem contere ; tum colocynthidem in pulverem tenuissimum tritam. et
oleum admisce, denique cum syrupo simplici subige in massam.

PILULÆ ALOES ET MYRRHÆ.

℞. Aloes socotrinæ uncias duas.
 Myrrhæ unciam unam.
 Croci unciam dimidiam.

Cum syrupo subige in massam.

PILLS.

ALOETIC PILLS.

Take of Socotrine aloes in powder.
Castile Soap each an equal part.

With water form a mass fit for making pills.

PILLS OF ALOES AND COLOCYNTH.

FORMERLY " PILULÆ COCHIÆ."

Take of Socotrine aloes ;
Scammony, each two ounces.
Sulphate of potass, two drachms.
Colocynth, an ounce.
Oil of cloves, two fluidrachms.

Reduce the aloes and scammony into a powder with the sulphate of potass, then add the colocynth in fine powder, and the oil of cloves, and with simple syrup form a mass.

PILLS OF ALOES AND MYRRH.

FORMERLY " PILULÆ RUFI."

Take of Socotrine aloes, two ounces.
Myrrh, one ounce.
Saffron, half an ounce.

Beat them into a mass with syrup

PILULÆ ALOES CUM MYRRHA ET GUAIACO.

℞. Aloes socotrinæ in pulverem tritæ unciam dimidiam.
Croci in pulverem triti ;
Myrrhæ in pulverem tritæ, utriusque drachmas duas.
Guaiaci resinæ in pulverem tritæ unciam dimidiam.
Oxidi antimonii unciam dimidiam.

Cum copaibâ subige in massam.

PILULÆ ANTIMONIALES COMPOSITÆ.

℞. Hydrargyri submuriatis drachmas duas.
Opii in pulverem triti drachmam unam.
Antimonii tartarizati scrupulum unum.

Cum syrupo subige in massam, et in pilulas sexaginta divide.

PILULÆ ARSENICI.

℞. Acidi arseniosi grana duo.
Opii in pulverem triti grana octo.
Saponis grana viginti duo.

Subige in massam, et divide in pilulas triginta duas.

PILULÆ ASSAFŒTIDÆ.

℞ Assafœtidæ partes tres.
Saponis partem unam.

Cum aqua subigantur in massam.

PILLS OF ALOES MYRRH AND GUAIACUM.

Take of Socotrine aloes in powder, half an ounce.
Saffron in powder ;
Myrrh in powder, each two drachms.
Resin of guaiacum in powder, half an ounce.
Oxide of antimony, half an ounce.

With copaiba form a mass.

COMPOUND ANTIMONIAL PILLS.

Take of Submuriate of mercury, two drachms.
Opium in powder, one drachm.
Tartarized antimony, one scruple.

With syrup form a mass to be divided into sixty pills.

PILLS OF ARSENIC.

Take of Arsenious acid, two grains.
Opium in powder, eight grains.
Castile soap, twenty-two grains.

Form a mass and divide into thirty-two pills.

ASSAFŒTIDA PILLS.

Take of Assafœtida, three parts.
Castile soap, one part.

With water beat into a mass.

23

PILULÆ ASSAFŒTIDÆ COMPOSITÆ.

℞. Assafœtidæ ;
   Aloes socotrinæ ;
   Saponis ; singulorum partem æqualem.

Cum aquâ subigantur in massam.

———

PILULÆ AURI MURIATIS.

℞. Auri muriatis grana decem.
   Glycyrrhizæ in pulverem tritæ drachmas tres.

Cum syrupo simplici subige in massam et divide in pilulas centum et quinquaginta.

———

PILULÆ COLOCYNTHIDIS EXTRACTI COMPO-SITI.

℞. Colocynthidis extracti compositi drachmam cum se-misse.
   Antimonii oxidi drachmam dimidiam.

Fiat massa, in pilulas triginta dividenda.

———

PILULÆ FERRI SULPHATIS.

℞ Ferri sulphatis drachmam unam.

Cum extracto gentianæ subige in massam et divide in pilulas triginta æquales.

COMPOUND ASSAFŒTIDA PILLS.

Take of Assafœtida ;
    Socotrine aloes ;
    Castile soap, each equal parts.

With water beat into a mass.

PILLS OF MURIATE OF GOLD.

Take of Muriate of gold, ten grains.
    Liquorice in powder, three drachms.

With simple syrup form a mass and divide into a hundred and fifty pills.

PILLS OF COMPOUND EXTRACT OF COLO-CYNTH.

Take of Compound extract of colocynth, a drachm and a half.
    Oxide of antimony, half a drachm.

Form a mass, and divide into thirty pills.

PILLS OF SULPHATE OF IRON.

Take of Sulphate of iron, one drachm.

With the extract of gentian form a mass, and divide into thirty pills.

PILULÆ FERRI SULPHATIS COMPOSITÆ.

℞. Rhei in pulverem triti drachmam cum semisse.
Ferri sulphatis scrupulos duos.
Saponis drachmam dimidiam.

Cum aquâ subige in massam et divide in pilulas quadraginta æquales.

PILULÆ GAMBOGIÆ ET SCAMMONIÆ.

℞. Gambogiæ in pulverem tritæ unciam unam.
Scammonii in pulverem triti unciam dimidiam.
Potassæ nitratis drachmam unam.
Saponis drachmas duas.

Cum aquâ subige in massam et divide in pilulas quadringentas.

PILULÆ HYDRARGYRI.

℞. Hydrargyri purificati ;
Confectionis rosæ, utriusque unciam unam.
Glycyrrhizæ in pulverem tritæ unciam dimidiam.

Tere hydrargyrum cum confectione in mortario vitreo donec illius globuli visum penitus effugerint ; dein glycyrrhizam adjice et subige in massam statim dividendam in pilulas quadringentas octoginta æquales.

PILULÆ HYDRARGYRI OXYMURIATIS.

℞. Hydrargyri oxymuriatis grana decem.
Marantæ scrupulum unum.

Cum ammoniæ muriate in aqua soluto subige in massam.

COMPOUND PILLS OF SULPHATE OF IRON.

Take of Rhubarb in powder, one drachm and a half.
    Sulphate of iron, two scruples.
    Castile soap, half a drachm.

With water form a mass and divide into forty pills.

PILLS OF GAMBOGE AND SCAMMONY.

Take of Gamboge in powder, one ounce.
    Scammony in powder, half an ounce.
    Nitrate of potass, one drachm.
    Castile soap, two drachms.

With water form a mass and divide into four hundred pills.

MERCURIAL PILLS.

BLUE PILLS.

Take of Purified mercury ;
    Confection of roses, each one ounce.
    Liquorice in powder, half an ounce.

Rub the mercury with the confection in a glass mortar till the globules disappear ; then add the liquorice and form a mass to be immediately divided into four hundred and eighty pills.

PILLS OF OXYMURIATE OF MERCURY.

Take of Oxymuriate of mercury, ten grains.
    Arrow root, one scruple.

With muriate of ammonia dissolved in water form a mass.

PILULÆ HYDRARGYRI SUBMURIATIS.

℞. Hydrargyri submuriatis drachmam dimidiam.
  Saponis scrupulum unum.

Cum aquâ subige in massam, et divide in pilulas triginta
æquales.

PILULÆ JALAPÆ COMPOSITÆ.

℞. Jalapæ in pulverem tritæ ;
  Rhei in pulverem triti ;
  Saponis, singulorum unciam unam.
  Hydrargyri submuriatis drachmas sex cum scrupulis
  duobus.
  Antimonii tartarizati grana viginti octo.

Cum aquâ subige in massam et divide in pilulas quadringentas
æquales.

PILULÆ MYRRHÆ ET FERRI.

℞. Ferri limaturæ purificatæ unciam unam.
  Myrrhæ in pulverem tritæ ;
  Saponis, utriusque drachmas duas.

Cum syrupo subige in massam et divide in pilulas singulas
grana sex pendentes.

PILULÆ OPII.

℞. Opii in pulverem triti drachmam unam.
  Saponis grana duodecim.

Cum aquâ subige in massam et divide in pilulas sexaginta
æquales.

PILLS OF SUBMURIATE OF MERCURY.

Take of Submuriate of mercury, half a drachm.
Castile soap, one scruple.

With water form a mass and divide into thirty pills.

COMPOUND PILLS OF JALAP.

Take of Jalap in powder ;
Rhubarb in powder ;
Castile soap, each one ounce.
Submuriate of mercury six drachms and two scruples.
Tartarized antimony, twenty eight grains.

With water form a mass and divide into four hundred pills.

PILLS OF MYRRH AND IRON.

Take of Purified iron filings, one ounce.
Myrrh in powder ;
Castile soap, each two drachms.

With syrup form a mass and divide into pills, each weighing six grains.

PILLS OF OPIUM.

Take of Opium in powder, one drachm.
Castile soap, twelve grains.

With water form a mass and divide into sixty pills.

PILULÆ PICIS.

℞. Picis liquidæ drachmam unam.

Inulæ in pulverem tritæ quantum sufficit ad forman-
dam massam in pilulas sexaginta dividendam.

PILULÆ RHEI COMPOSITÆ.

℞. Rhei in pulverem triti unciam unam.
Aloës socotrinæ in pulverem tritæ drachmas sex.
Myrrhæ in pulverem tritæ unciam dimidiam.
Olei menthæ piperitæ fluidrachmam dimidiam.

Cum syrupo aurantii corticis subige in massam.

PILULÆ SCILLÆ.

℞. Scillæ siccatæ in pulverem tritæ drachmam unam.
Saponis grana viginti quatuor.

Cum aquâ subige in massam et divide in pilulas quadraginta
æquales.

PILULÆ SODÆ SUBCARBONATIS.

℞. Sodæ subcarbonatis exsiccatæ drachmas duas.
Saponis drachmam dimidiam.

Subige in massam et divide in pilulas quadraginta æquales.

TAR PILLS.

Take of Tar one drachm.

Elecampane in powder, a sufficient quantity to form a mass to be divided into sixty pills.

COMPOUND PILLS OF RHUBARB.

Take of Rhubarb in powder, one ounce.
Socotrine aloes in powder, six drachms.
Myrrh in powder, half an ounce.
Oil of peppermint, half a fluidrachm.

With syrup of orange peel, form a mass.

PILLS OF SQUILL.

Take of Dried squills in powder, one drachm.
Castile soap, twenty-four grains.

With water form a mass, and divide into forty pills.

PILLS OF SUBCARBONATE OF SODA.

Take of Subcarbonate of soda, dried, two drachms.
Castile soap, half a drachm.

Form a mass, and divide into forty pills.

24

PLUMBUM.

PLUMBI ACETAS.

℞. Plumbi subcarbonatis quantumvis.
Aceti purificati pondus decuplum.

Digere in vase vitreo, donec dulcescat acetum.   Tum hoc effuso, aceti perge addens donec non amplius dulcescat.   Cola, et alternatim lente vaporando et refrigerando, in crystallos redige sub umbra exsiccandas.

PLUMBI SUBACETAS LIQUIDUS.

℞. Plumbi oxidi semivitrei libras duas.
Aceti purificati congium unum.

Misce, et decoque ad octantes sex, assiduè movens ; dein sepone, ut subsidant fæces, et cola.

POTASSA.

POTASSA.

℞. Aquæ potassæ quantumvis.

In vase ferreo mundissimo operto vaporet, donec, ebullitione finitâ, materies salina tranquillè fluat instar olei, quod fit ante

LEAD.

ACETATE OF LEAD.

SUGAR OF LEAD.

Take of Subcarbonate of lead, any quantity.
Purified vinegar, ten times its weight.

Digest in a glass vessel until the vinegar becomes sweet. Having poured this off, add more vinegar, until it ceases to become sweet. Filter the liquor and crystallize by alternate slow evaporation and refrigeration. The crystals are to be dried in the shade.

LIQUID SUBACETATE OF LEAD.

GOULARD'S EXTRACT.

Take of Semivitrified oxide of lead, two pounds.
Purified vinegar, one gallon.

Mix, and boil down to six pints, constantly stirring ; then set it by, that the feculencies may subside, and strain.

POTASS.

POTASS.

Take of Solution of potass, any quantity.

Evaporate it in a covered very clean iron vessel, till, on the ebullition ceasing, the saline matter flows gently like oil, which

quam vas igne rubescat. Dein effundatur super laminam ferream nitidam ; in massulas secetur antequam durescat, et illico in phiala bene obturanda reponatur.

POTASSÆ ACETAS.

℞. Potassæ carbonatis libram unam.

Coquatur, lenissimo igne, in aceti purificati quadruplo vel quintuplo ; et denuo acetum subinde adjiciatur, donec prioris parte aquosâ fere vaporando dissipatâ, acetum nuper additum nullam moveat effervescentiam, quod fiet consumptis aceti octantibus circiter viginti ; postea lentè exsiccetur. Sal impurus residuus, leni igne aliquantisper, nec justo diutius, liquefiat ; dein aquâ solvatur, et per chartam coletur. Si liquefactio rite peracta fuerit, liquor colatus limpidus erit, sin minus, coloris fusci. Postea, lenissimo igne vaporet hic liquor ex vase vitreo minime profundo, sale, dum arescit, subinde moto, quo citius ad siccitatem perducatur. Acetas potassæ dein in vase optime clauso asservari debet, ne aëre liquescat.

AQUA POTASSÆ.

℞. Calcis recentis uncias octo.
Potassæ carbonatis uncias sex.

Injiciatur calx in vas ferreum vel figulinum, cum aquæ calidæ fluidunciis viginti octo. Ebullitione peractâ, statim addatur sal ; omnibusque bene permistis, vas operiatur donec frigescant. Frigefacta materia, et dein bene agitata, effundatur in infundibulum vitreum, cujus guttur linteolo puro obstructum sit. Infundi-

happens before the vessel becomes red. Then pour it out on a smooth iron plate ; let it be divided into small pieces before it hardens, and immediately deposited in a well-stopped phial.

ACETATE OF POTASS.

FORMERLY DIURETIC SALT.

Take of Carbonate of potass, one pound.

Boil it with a very gentle heat in four or five times its weight of purified vinegar, and add more vinegar at different times, till on the watery part of the preceding quantity being nearly dissipated by evaporation, the new addition of vinegar ceases to raise any effervescence, which will happen when about twenty pints of vinegar have been consumed. It is then to be slowly dried. The impure salt remaining is to be melted with a gentle heat, for a short time, but no longer than necessary, and afterwards dissolved in water, and filtered through paper. If the liquefaction has been properly performed, the filtered liquor will be limpid ; but if otherwise, of a brown colour. Afterwards evaporate this liquor with a very gentle heat, in a very shallow glass vessel, occasionally stirring the salt as it becomes dry, that its moisture may be sooner dissipated. Lastly, the acetate of potass ought to be kept in a vessel very closely stopped, to prevent it from deliquescing.

SOLUTION OF POTASS.

Take of Fresh burnt lime, eight ounces.
Carbonate of potass, six ounces.

Put the lime into an iron or earthen vessel, with twenty-eight fluidounces of warm water. After the ebullition is finished, instantly add the salt ; and having thoroughly mixed them, cover the vessel till they cool. When the mixture has cooled, agitate it well, and pour it into a glass funnel, the throat of which is stopped with a piece of clean linen. Cover the upper ori-

buli os superius operiatur dum tubus ejus alii vasi vitreo insera-
tur, ut aqua potassæ per linteolum in vas suppositum sensim
stillet. Cùm primum stillare desiêrit, affundantur in infundibulum aquæ fluidunciæ aliquot, sed cautè, ut ea materiam supernatet. Incipiet iterum stillare aqua potassæ. Sic autem iteranda
est aquæ affusio, donec stillaverint octantes tres, quod bidui vel
tridui spatio fiet ; dein liquoris partes superiores cum inferiori-
bus agitatione misceantur ; ipseque in vase bène obturato servetur

---

POTASSÆ CARBONAS.

℞. Potassæ supertartratis quantumvis.

Charta bibulâ madefactâ involutus, vel crucibulo inditus, cir-
cumjectis prunis, in massam nigram comburatur ; quæ dein con-
trita in crucibulo aperto, igni mediocri subjiciatur usque donec
alba vel saltem cinerea fiat ; curâ adhibitâ ne liquescat. Tum
in aqua calida solvatur ; per linteum coletur liquor, et in vase
ferreo mundo vaporet, sub finem assidue agitatus cochleari ferreo ne materia fundo vasis adhæreat. Sal albissimus restabit,
qui paulo diutius super ignem relinquendus est, donec vasis fundus fere rubescat. Postremo refrigeratus in vasis vitreis. bene
obturatis servetur.

POTASSA CUM CALCE.

℞. Aquæ potassæ quantumvis.

Vaporet ad tertiam partem in vase ferreo operto ; dein ad-
misceatur calcis recèns extinctæ quantum sufficiat ad pultis so-
lidioris crassitudinem dandam, quæ in vase obturato servetur.

fice of the funnel, and insert its tube into another glass vessel,
so that the solution of potass may gradually drop through the
rag into the lower vessel. As soon as it ceases to drop, pour
into the funnel some ounces of water, but cautiously, so that it
may swim above the matter in the funnel. The solution of potass will again begin to drop, and the effusion of water is to be
repeated in the same manner, until three pints have dropped,
which will happen in the space of two or three days ; then mix
the superior and inferior parts of the liquor together by agitation, and keep it in a well-stopped phial.

CARBONATE OF POTASS.

Take of Impure supertartrate of potass, any quantity.

Wrap it up in moist bibulous paper, or put it into a crucible,
and burn it into a black mass, by placing it among live coals.
Having reduced this mass to powder, expose it in an open crucible to the action of a moderate fire, till it become white, or at
least of an ash-grey colour, taking care that it do not melt. Then
dissolve it in warm water ; strain the liquor through a linen
cloth, and evaporate it in a clean iron vessel, diligently stirring it towards the end of the process, with an iron spatula,
to prevent it from sticking to the bottom of the vessel. A very
white salt will remain, which is to be left a little longer on the
fire, till the bottom of the vessel becomes almost red. Lastly,
when the salt is grown cold, keep it in glass vessels well stopped.

POTASS WITH LIME.

Take of Solution of potass, any quantity.

Evaporate it in a covered iron vessel till one third remains ;
then mix it with as much new slacked lime as will bring it to the
consistence of pretty solid pap, which is to be kept in a vessel
closely stopped.

POTASSÆ SUBCARBONAS.

℞. Potassæ subcarbonatis impuri quantumvis.

·In crucibulo igne rubescat, dein cum aquâ pari pondere contere et postquam subsederint fæces, liquorem in ollam ferream
mundissimam infunde ; denique ad siccitatem decoque sub finem,
assidue, ne vasi adhæreat, agitans.

LIQUOR POTASSÆ SUBCARBONATIS.

℞. Potassæ subcarbonatis libram unam.
Aquæ distillatæ fluiduncias duodecim.

Liqua potassæ subcarbonatem in aquâ, et per chartam cola.

POTASSÆ SULPHAS.

℞. Salis qui restat post distillationem acidi nitrici, libras
duas.
Aquæ bullientis congios duos.

Misce, ut liquetur sal ; tum adjice potassæ subcarbonatis quod
satis sit ad acidum saturandum. Dein coque, donec pellicula
supernatet, et, postquam colaveris, sepone, ut fiant crystalli.
Has, effusâ aquâ, super chartam bibulam exsicca.

SUBCARBONATE OF POTASS.

FORMERLY SALT OF TARTAR.

Take of Impure subcarbonate of potass, any quantity.

Heat it red hot in a crucible. Then triturate it with an equal weight of water, and after the fæces have subsided, pour the liquor into a very clean iron pot ; lastly, boil to dryness, stirring constantly towards the end of the process, to prevent it from sticking to the vessel.

SOLUTION OF SUBCARBONATE OF POTASS.

Take of Subcarbonate of potass, one pound.
Distilled water, twelve fluidounces.

Dissolve the subcarbonate of potass in the water, and then strain the solution through paper.

SULPHATE OF POTASS.

FORMERLY VITRIOLATED TARTAR.

Take of Salt which remains after the distillation of nitric acid, two pounds.
Boiling water, two gallons.

Mix them together that the salt may be dissolved ; next add as much subcarbonate of potass as may be requisite for the saturation of the acid. Then boil the solution until a pellicle appears upon the surface, and, after straining it, set it by that crystals may form. Having poured away the water, dry the crystals upon bibulous paper.

25

POTASSÆ SUPERCARBONAS.

R. Potassæ carbonatis partem unam.
Aquæ partes tres.

Solve in aqua potassæ carbonatem. Liquorem in vas Noothii apparatus medium pone ; et per idem, acidum carbonicum a calcis carbonate et acido sulphurico diluto elicitum, donec crystallos deponere cessaverit, transire facias ; dein crystallos collige, et super charta bibula exsicca.

POTASSÆ TARTRAS.

R. Potassæ subcarbonatis libram unam.
Potassæ supertartratis libras tres, vel quantum satis sit.
Aquæ bullientis octantes quindecim.

Potassæ subcarbonati in aqua soluto potassæ supertartratem in pulverem tenuem tritum paulatim adjice, quamdiu effervescentiam excitet, quæ fere desinit antequam triplum subcarbonatis potassæ pondus injectum fuerit ; dein liquorem refrigeratum per chartam cola, et post idoneam exhalationem sepone ut crystalli formentur.

TARTRAS POTASSÆ ET SODÆ.

R. Sodæ subcarbonatis uncias viginti.
Potassæ supertartratis contritæ libras duas.
Aquæ bullientis octantes decem.

Sodæ subcarbonatem in aquâ liqua, et adjice paulatim potassæ supertartratem. Liquorem per chartam cola ; tum coque, donec pellicula supernatet, et sepone, ut fiant crystalli. Has, effusâ aquâ, super chartam bibulam exsicca.

SUPER-CARBONATE OF POTASS.

Take of Carbonate of potass, one part.
Water, three parts.

Dissolve the carbonate of potass in the water; put the solution in the middle vessel of Nooth's apparatus, and pass through it a stream of carbonic acid gas, obtained from carbonate of lime and diluted sulphuric acid, until the deposition of crystals ceases; then collect the crystals, and dry them on bibulous paper.

TARTRATE OF POTASS.
FORMERLY SOLUBLE TARTAR.

Take of Subcarbonate of potass, one pound.
Supertartrate of potass, three pounds, or as much as may be sufficient.
Boiling water, fifteen pints.

To the subcarbonate of potass, dissolved in the water, gradually add the supertartrate of potass in fine powder, as long as it raises any effervescence, which generally ceases before three times the weight of the subcarbonate of potass has been added; then strain the cooled liquor through paper; and, after due evaporation, set it aside to crystallize.

TARTRATE OF POTASS AND SODA.
CALLED ROCHELLE SALT.

Take of Subcarbonate of soda, twenty ounces.
Supertartrate of potass in powder, two pounds.
Boiling water, ten pints.

Dissolve the carbonate of soda in the water, and gradually add the supertartrate of potass. Filter the solution through paper; evaporate until a pellicle be formed, and set it aside to crystallize. Pour off the liquor, and dry the crystals on blotting paper.

PULVERES.

PULVIS ALOES CUM CANELLA.

℞. Aloës socotrinæ libram unam.
Canellæ uncias tres.

Separatim in pulverem tenuissimum tere ; dein misce.

PULVIS AROMATICUS.

℞. Cinnamomi ;
Cardamomi ;
Zingiberis ; singulorum partem æqualem.

Tere in pulverem tenuissimum, qui in vase vitreo bene obturato servandus est.

PULVIS CALCIS CARBONATIS COMPOSITUS.

℞. Calcis carbonatis præparati uncias quatuor.
Cinnamomi drachmam unam cum semisse.
Myristicæ drachmam dimidiam.

Tere simul in pulverem.

PULVIS IPECACUANHÆ ET CUPRI SULPHATIS.

℞. Ipecacuanhæ in pulverem tritæ scrupulum unum.
Cupri sulphatis grana quinque.

Tere simul in pulverem.

POWDERS.

POWDER OF ALOES WITH CANELLA.
FORMERLY "HIERA PICRA."

Take of Socotrine aloes, one pound.
    Canella, three ounces.

Pulverize them separately ; then mix them.

AROMATIC POWDER.

Take of Cinnamon ;
    Cardamon ;
    Ginger, each equal parts.

Rub them together to a fine powder, which is to be kept in a
well stopped glass bottle.

COMPOUND POWDER OF CARBONATE OF LIME.

Take of Prepared carbonate of lime, four ounces.
    Cinnamon, a drachm and a half.
    Nutmeg, half a drachm.

Powder them together.

POWDER OF IPECACUANHA AND SULPHATE OF COPPER.

Take of Ipecacuanha in powder, one scruple.
    Sulphate of copper, five grains.

Rub them together.

PULVIS IPECACUANHÆ ET OPII.

R. Ipecacuanhæ in pulverem tritæ.
Opii, utriusque partem unam.
Potassæ sulphatis partes octo.

Tere simul in pulverem tenuem.

PULVIS JALAPÆ COMPOSITUS

R. Jalapæ in pulverem tritæ partem unam.
Potassæ supertartratis partes duas.

Tere simul in pulverem tenuissimum.

PULVIS SCAMMONII COMPOSITUS.

R. Scammonii
Potassæ supertartratis, utriusque partem æqualem.

Tere simul in pulverem tenuissimum.

SODA.

SODÆ CARBONAS.

R. Sodæ subcarbonatis libram unam.
Ammoniæ subcarbonatis uncias tres.
Aquæ distillatæ octantem unum.

Sodæ subcarbonati in aquâ liquato ammoniam adjice ; tum
balneo arenæ caloris gradum clxxx, adhibe per horas tres, vel

POWDER OF IPECACUANHA AND OPIUM.

FORMERLY DOVER'S POWDER.

Take of Ipecacuanha, in powder ;
  Opium, each one part.
  Sulphate of potass, eight parts.

Reduce them to a fine powder.

———

COMPOUND POWDER OF JALAP.

Take of Jalap in powder, one part.
  Supertartrate of potass, two parts.

Rub them together to a fine powder.

———

COMPOUND POWDER OF SCAMMONY.

Take of Scammony ;
  Supertartrate of potass, each equal parts.

Rub them together to a fine powder.

———

SODA.

CARBONATE OF SODA.

Take of Subcarbonate of soda, one pound.
  Carbonate of ammonia, three ounces.
  Water, one pint.

Having previously dissolved the subcarbonate of soda in the water, add the carbonate of ammonia, then by means of a sand

donec ammonia expulsa fuerit. Denique sepone, ut fiant crystalli. Simili modo consumatur liquor reliquus, et seponatur, ut
iterum prodeant crystalli.

SODÆ PHOSPHAS.

℞. Phosphatis calcis in pulverem contusi libras decem.
Acidi sulphurici libras sex.
Aquæ octantes novem
Subcarbonatis sodæ quantum satis sit.

Phosphatem calcis in vase figulino cum acido sulphurico permisce ; dein adde aquam et iterum permisce ; tunc vas in aquæ
bullientis vapore fove per tres dies, quibus elapsis, materiam
aliis aquæ bullientis octantibus novem additis dilue, et per pan-
num linteum fortem cola, aquam bullientem paulatim superin-
fundens, donec acidum omne eluatur. Liquorem colatum sepone, ut fæces subsidant, a quibus effunde ; dein vaporatione
minue ad octantes novem. Huic liquori a fæcibus effuso, et
calefacto in vase figulino, adde subcarbonatem sodæ ex aqua calida solutum, donec cesset effervescentia. Tum cola, et sepone,
ut crystalli formentur. His exemptis, liquori, si opus sit, adde
paululum subcarbonatis sodæ, ut acidum phosphoricum accuratè
saturetur, et vaporatione ad crystallos iterum formandos dis-
pone, quamdiu hi prodierint. Crystalli demum in vase bene
obturando reponantur.

SODÆ MURIAS EXSICCATUS.

℞. Sodæ muriatis quantumvis.

Super ignem torre in vase ferreo, minus arcte cooperto, su-
hinde agitans, donec crepitare cessaverit.

bath apply a heat of 180° for three hours, or until the ammonia be driven off. Lastly, set the solution by to crystallize. The remaining solution may in the same manner be evaporated and set by, that crystals may again form.

PHOSPHATE OF SODA.

Take of Phosphate of lime in coarse powder, ten pounds.
  Sulphuric acid, six pounds.
  Water, nine pints.
  Subcarbonate of soda, a sufficient quantity.

Mix the phosphate of lime with the sulphuric acid in an earthen vessel ; then add the water, and mix again ; then place the vessel in a vapour bath, and digest for three days ; after which, dilute the mass with nine pints more of boiling water, and strain the liquor through a strong linen cloth, pouring over it boiling water in small quantities at a time, until the whole acid be washed out. Set by the strained liquor, that the impurities may subside ; decant the clear solution, and evaporate it to nine pints. To this liquor poured from the impurities, and heated in an earthen vessel, add carbonate of soda, dissolved in warm water, until the effervescence ceases. Filter the neutralized liquor, and set it aside to crystallize. To the liquor that remains after the crystals are taken out add a little carbonate of soda, if necessary, so as to saturate exactly the phosphoric acid ; and dispose the liquor, by evaporation, to form crystals as long as it will furnish any. Lastly, the crystals are to be kept in a wellclosed vessel.

DRIED MURIATE OF SODA.

Take of Muriate of soda, any quantity.

Roast it over the fire in an iron vessel, loosely covered, until it ceases to decrepitate, agitating it from time to time.

SODÆ SUBCARBONAS EXSICCATUS.

℞. Sodæ subcarbonatis quantumvis.

In vase ferreo nitido, calorem ferventem adhibe, donec penitus exsiccetur; simul spathâ ferreâ assiduè movens. Denique in pulverem tere.

SPIRITUS.

SPIRITUS JUNIPERI COMPOSITUS.

℞. Juniperi contusæ libram unam.
    Carui contusi;
    Fæniculi contusi, utriusque unciam unam cum semisse.
    Alcoholis diluti octantes novem.

Macera per biduum; et addito aquæ quantum satis sit ad arcendum empyreuma, distillatione elice octantes novem.

SPIRITUS LAVANDULÆ.

℞. Lavandulæ recentis libras duas.
    Alcoholis congium unum.

Macera per horas viginti quatuor; et addito aquæ quantum satis sit ad arcendum empyreuma, distillatione elice congium.

SPIRITUS RORISMARINI.

℞. Rorismarini recentis libras duas.
    Alcoholis congium unum.

Macera per biduum; et addito aquæ quantum satis sit ad arcendum empyreuma distillatione elice congium.

DRIED SUBCARBONATE OF SODA.

Take of Subcarbonate of soda, any quantity.

Apply to it a boiling heat in a clean iron vessel until it becomes perfectly dry, and at the same time constantly stir it with an iron rod. Lastly, reduce it to powder.

SPIRITS.

COMPOUND SPIRIT OF JUNIPER.

Take of Juniper bruised, one pound.
  Caraway bruised ;
  Fennel bruised, each one ounce and a half.
  Diluted alcohol, nine pints.

Macerate for two days ; and having added enough water to prevent empyreuma, distil off nine pints.

SPIRIT OF LAVENDER.

Take of Fresh lavender, two pounds.
  Alcohol, one gallon.

Macerate for twenty hours ; and having added enough water to prevent empyreuma, distil off a gallon.

SPIRIT OF ROSEMARY.

Take of Fresh rosemary, two pounds.
  Alcohol, one gallon.

Macerate for twenty-four hours, and having added enough water to prevent empyreuma, distil off a gallon.

SPONGIA.

SPONGIA USTA.

R. Spongiæ quantumvis.

In frustula concide, et contunde, ut a rebus alienis adhærentibus separetur ; tum in vase ferreo clauso ure, donec nigra et friabilis fiat ; denique in pulverem subtilissimum tere.

STANNUM.

PULVIS STANNI.

R. Stanni quantumvis.

Liqua in vase ferreo super ignem, et agita donec in pulverem redactum fuerit ; quem refrigeratum per cribrum transmitte.

PULVIS STANNI AMALGAMATIS.

R Stanni partes quinque.
Hydrargyri purificati partes duas.
Calcis carbonatis præparati partem unam.

Stanno liquefacto hydrargyrum adde, et simul contere ; tum carbonate calcis adjecto, misturam adhuc liquentem, donec particulæ metallicæ evanuerint, tere. Inter frigescendum misturam in pollen redige.

SPONGE.

BURNT SPONGE.

Take of Sponge, any quantity.

Cut it into pieces, and beat it, that any extraneous adherent matters may be separated ; then burn it in a close iron vessel until it becomes black and friable ; lastly rub it to a very fine powder.

TIN.

POWDER OF TIN.

Take of Tin, any quantity.

Having melted it over the fire in an iron vessel, agitate it until it be reduced to powder, which is to be passed, when cold, through a sieve.

POWDER OF THE AMALGAM OF TIN.

Take of Tin, five parts.
   Purified mercury, two parts.
   Prepared carbonate of lime, one part.

Melt the tin, add to it the mercury, and rub them together ; then add the carbonate of lime, and while the mixture is liquid, rub till the metallic particles disappear ; lastly, while the mixture cools, reduce it to an impalpable powder.

SULPHUREA.

SULPHURETUM POTASSÆ.

℞. Sulphuris unciam unam.
     Potassæ subcarbonatis uncias duas.

Simul contere, et in crucibulo clauso, super ignem lenem donec fusa sit mistura, retine.   Ex crucibulo adhuc calentem
funde ; et frigefactam in vase bene obturato serva.

SULPHURETUM SODÆ.

℞. Sulphuris ;
     Sodæ subcarbonatis exsiccati, utriusque unciam unam.

Modo eodem, quo potassæ sulphuretum, para.

SYRUPI.

SYRUPUS ACETI.

℞. Aceti purificati octantes duos cum semisse.
     Sacchari libras tres cum semisse.

Coque ut fiat syrupus.

SYRUPUS ALLII.

℞. Allii concisi libram unam.
     Aquæ bullientis octantes duos.

PREPARATIONS OF SULPHUR.

SULPHURET OF POTASS.

Take of Sulphur, one ounce.
> Subcarbonate of potass, two ounces.

Rub them together, and heat the mixture in a covered crucible, over a gentle fire, until it is fused.   Pour it from the crucible while hot, and after it has cooled, put it into a close stopped bottle.

SULPHURET OF SODA.

Take of Sulphur ;
> Dried subcarbonate of soda, of each, one ounce.

Prepare it in the same manner as sulphuret of potass.

SYRUPS.

SYRUP OF VINEGAR.

Take of Purified vinegar, two pints and a half.
> Sugar, three pounds and a half.

Boil them to form a syrup.

SYRUP OF GARLIC.

Take of Garlic sliced, one pound.
> Boiling water, two pints.

Macera allium in aqua, vase operto, per horas duodecim, dein liquoris colati parti uni adjice sacchari partes duas, et fiat syrupus.

SYRUPUS AURANTII CORTICIS.

R. Aurantii corticis exterioris recentis uncias tres.
Aquæ bullientis octantem unum cum semisse.
Sacchari libras tres.

Digere corticem in aqua per horas duodecim vase operto, vesiculas radula discerpens ; dein liquori colato adde saccharum contritum, leni calore adhibito, ut fiat syrupus.

SYRUPUS COLCHICI.

R. Colchici recentis in frustra tenuia secti unciam unam.
Aceti purificati octantem unum.
Sacchari uncias viginti sex.

Macera colchicum in aceto per biduum, vas subinde agitans, dein leniter exprimens cola. Liquori colato adde saccharum contritum, et coque paululum ut fiat syrupus.

SYRUPUS RHAMNI.

R. Succi defæcati baccarum maturarum rhamni partes duas.
Sacchari partem unam.

Coque ut fiat syrupus.

Macerate the garlic in the water, in a covered vessel, for twelve hours ; then add two parts of sugar, to one part of the strained liquor, and form a syrup.

SYRUP OF ORANGE PEEL.

Take of Fresh orange peel, three ounces.
    Boiling water, one pint and a half.
    Sugar, three pounds.

Digest for twelve hours in a covered vessel, during which time, lacerate the oil vesicles under water by rubbing a grater upon the outside of the peel ; then add to the strained liquor the sugar in powder, and with a very gentle heat form a syrup.

SYRUP OF MEADOW SAFFRON.

Take of Fresh meadow saffron cut in slices, one ounce
    Purified vinegar, one pint.
    Sugar, twenty-six ounces.

Macerate the meadow saffron in the vinegar for two days, occasionally shaking the vessel ; then strain the infusion with gentle expression. To the strained infusion add the sugar ; and boil a little so as to form a syrup.

SYRUP OF BUCKTHORN.

Take of Defecated juice of ripe buckthorn, two parts.
    Sugar, one part.

Boil to form a syrup.

SYRUPUS RHEI.

℞. Rhei contusi uncias duas.
Aquæ bullientis octantem unum.

Macera per horas viginti quatuor, cola, et adde liquoris parti
uni sacchari partes duas ; dein ut fiat syrupus, coque.

SYRUPUS RHEI AROMATICUS.

℞. Rhei contusi drachmas quinque.
Caryophyllorum ;
Cinnamomi, utriusque unciam dimidiam.
Myristicæ nucleos duos.
Aquæ octantem unum.

Digere et vaporet, donec liquor ad octantem dimidium sit redactus ; cola, et libram sacchari unam, et octantem dimidium alcoholis diluti adde. Dein coque paulisper, ut fiat syrupus.

SYRUPUS RHEI CUM SENNA.

℞. Rhei contusi ;
Sennæ, utriusque unciam unam cum semisse.
Cardamomi drachmas tres.
Aquæ ferventis octantem unum.

Digere per horas viginti quatuor ; tum calore leni, donec ad
octantem dimidium redactus sit liquor, vaporet ; dein cola, et
adde sacchari libram unam ; denique, ut fiat syrupus, coque.

SYRUP OF RHUBARB.

Take of Rhubarb bruised, two ounces.
Boiling water, one pint.

Macerate for twenty-four hours ; strain, and add two parts of sugar to one of the liquor ; then boil to form a syrup.

AROMATIC SYRUP OF RHUBARB.

Take of Rhubarb bruised, five drachms.
Cloves ;
Cinnamon, each half an ounce.
Nutmegs, two in number.
Water, one pint.

Digest and evaporate till the liquor is reduced to half a pint ; strain, and add one pound of sugar, and half a pint of diluted alcohol ; then boil a little to form a syrup.

SYRUP OF RHUBARB WITH SENNA.

Take of Rhubarb, bruised ;
Senna, each one ounce and a half.
Cardamom, three drachms.
Boiling water, one pint.

Digest for twenty-four hours, and evaporate with a gentle heat till the liquor is reduced to half a pint ; then strain and add one pound of sugar ; lastly boil to form a syrup.

SYRUPUS SARSAPARILLÆ.

℞. Sarsaparillæ concisæ libras duas.
Glycyrrhizæ concisæ ;
Rosæ ;
Sennæ ;
Anisi singulorum uncias duas.
Aquæ tepidæ octantes duodecim.

Macera sarsaparillam per horas viginti quatuor in aqua
dein coque per horæ quadrantem ; et valide exprimens cola.
Bulliat denuo sarsaparilla cum aquæ decem octantibus, vaporet-
que ad dimidium ; tum cola, et liquores mistos additis cæteris
coque iterum ad dimidium consumendum. Cola, et adde

Mellis despumati ;
Sacchari, utriusque libras duas.

Coque in syrupum densiorem.

SYRUPUS SARSAPARILLÆ ET GUAIACI.

℞. Sarsaparillæ concisæ ;
Guaiaci rasi, utriusque libram unam.
Rosæ ;
Acaciæ gummi :
Sennæ, uniuscujusque unciam unam.
Zingiberis unciam dimidiam.
Aquæ octantes decem.

Coque sarsaparillam et guaiacum in aqua, horam unam ; cola,
et residuo aquæ octantes alteros decem, adde ; coque denuo per horas duas, et sub finem bulliendi, rosam, acaciam,
sennam et zingiber adde ; cola, et decoctis adde mellis purificati, et sacchari, utriusque libras tres ; et, ut fiat syrupus, coque.

SYRUP•OF SARSAPARILLA.

Take of Sarsaparilla sliced, two pounds.
> Liquorice sliced ;
> Roses ;
> Senna ;
> Anise, each two ounces.
> Warm water, twelve pints.

Infuse the sarsaparilla in the water for twenty four hours , then boil for a quarter of an hour ; and strain by strong compression ; boil the sarsaparilla again in ten pints of water to the consumption of one half of the liquor ; strain, mix the two liquors, and add the other ingredients. Boil again to the consumption of one half of the liquor ; strain, and add of

> Honey ;
> Sugar, each two pounds.

Boil to form a thick syrup.

SYRUP OF SARSAPARILLA AND GUAIACUM.

Take of Sarsaparilla, sliced ;
> Guaiacum, rasped, of each one pound.
> Roses ;
> Acacia gum ;
> Senna, each one ounce.
> Ginger, half an ounce.
> Water, ten pints.

Boil the two first ingredients in the water for one hour, strain, and to the residuum add ten pints more of water ; boil for two hours and, towards the end of the boiling, add the other ingredients ; strain, and to the decoctions, add of clarified honey and sugar, each three pounds ; and boil to form a syrup

SYRUPUS SCILLÆ.

℞. Aceti scillæ octantes duos.
Sacchari contriti libras tres cum semisse.

Solvatur leni calore saccharum, ut fiat syrupus.

SYRUPUS SENEGÆ.

℞. Senegæ contusæ uncias quatuor.
Aquæ octantem unum.
Sacchari libram unam.

Coque senegam in aqua ad consumendam dimidiam. Laticem
purum transfunde ; saccharum adde ; et, donec fiat syrupus,
coque.

SYRUPUS SIMPLEX.

℞. Sacchari triti uncias quindecim.
Aquæ octantem dimidium.

Leni calore solvatur saccharum in aqua, et coquatur paululum,
ut, spuma ablata, fiat syrupus.

SYRUPUS TOLUTANI.

℞. Syrupi simplicis octantes duos.
Tincturæ tolutani fluidunciam unam.

Syrupo recèns parato, et ab igne remoto, cum pene refrixerit,
immisce paulatim tincturam, assiduè agitans.

SYRUP OF SQUILL.

Take of Vinegar of squill, two pints.
Sugar in powder, three pounds and a half,

Dissolve the sugar with a gentle heat so as to form a syrup.

SYRUP OF SENECA SNAKEROOT.

Take of Seneca snakeroot bruised, four ounces.
Water, one pint.
Sugar, one pound.

Boil the snakeroot in the water, to the consumption of the one half, decant the clear liquid, add the sugar, and boil to form a syrup.

SIMPLE SYRUP.

Take of Sugar in powder, fifteen ounces.
Water, half a pint.

Let the sugar be dissolved by a gentle heat in the water, and boiled a little, so as to form a syrup, the scum being removed.

SYRUP OF BALSAM OF TOLU.

Take of Simple syrup, two pints.
Tincture of tolu, one fluidounce.

With the syrup just prepared, and when it has almost grown cold, after having been removed from the fire, gradually mix the tincture with constant agitation.

SYRUPUS ZINGIBERIS.

R. Zingiberis in pulverem triti uncias tres.
Aquæ bullientis octantes quatuor.
Sacchari libras septem cum semisse.

Macera zingiber in aqua, vase clauso, per horas viginti quatuor ; dein liquori colato adde saccharum contritum, ut fiat syrupus.

TROCHISCI.

TROCHISCI GLYCYRRHIZÆ CUM OPIO.

R. Opii drachmas duas.
Tincturæ tolutani fluidunciam dimidiam.
Syrupi simplicis fluiduncias octo.
Glycyrrhizæ extracti aqua calida molliti.
Acaciæ gummi in pulverem triti, utriusque uncias
quinque.

Primum tere opium diligenter cum tinctura ; dein paulatim
admisce syrupum et extractum ; postea paulatim insperge pulverem acaciæ gummi, et tandem exsicca, ut fiat massa in trochiscos formanda, singulos grana decem pendentes.

TROCHISCI CALCIS CARBONATIS.

R. Calcis carbonatis præparati uncias quatuor.
Acaciæ gummi unciam unam.
Myristicæ drachmam unam.
Sacchari uncias sex.

Hæc in pulverem terantur et cum aqua fiat massa in trochiscos formanda.

SYRUP OF GINGER.

Take of Ginger in powder, three ounces.
    Boiling water, four pints.
    Sugar, seven pounds and a half.

Macerate the ginger in the water, in a close vessel, for twenty-four hours ; strain the infusion, add the sugar powdered, and form a syrup.

TROCHES.

TROCHES OF LIQUORICE AND OPIUM.

Take of Opium, two drachms.
    Tincture of tolu, half a fluidounce.
    Simple syrup, eight fluidounces.
    Extract of liquorice softened in hot water
    Acacia gum in powder, each five ounces.

First rub the opium thoroughly with the tincture, then by degrees add the syrup and extract ; after which, gradually sprinkle in the powdered gum, finally dry the mass, and form into troches, each weighing ten grains.

TROCHES OF CARBONATE OF LIME.

Take of Prepared carbonate of lime, four ounces.
    Acacia gum, one ounce.
    Nutmeg, one drachm.
    Sugar, six ounces.

Rub them into a powder, and form them by means of water, into a mass fit for making troches.

TROCHISCI MAGNESIÆ.

℞. Magnesiæ uncias quatuor.
Sacchari uncias duas.
Zingiberis in pulverem triti scrupulum unum.

Simul terantur, et cum syrupo simplici fiat massa in trochiscos formanda.

TINCTURÆ.

Digerantur tincturæ in vasis vitreis obturatis, calore circa gradum octogesimum, nisi aliter jussum fuerit. Inter parandum, sæpius agitari oportet.

TINCTURA ALOES.

℞. Aloes socotrinæ in pulverem tritæ unciam dimidiam.
Glycyrrhizæ extracti unciam unam cum semisse.
Alcoholis, fluiduncias quatuor.
Aquæ octantem unum.

Digere per dies decem, et tincturam defæcatam effunde.

TINCTURA ALOES ET MYRRHÆ.

℞. Myrrhæ in pulverem tritæ, uncias duas.
Alcoholis octantem unum cum semisse.
Aquæ octantem dimidium.

TROCHES OF MAGNESIA.

Take of Magnesia, four ounces.
    Sugar, two ounces.
    Ginger in powder, one scruple.

Rub them together, and, with simple syrup form them into a mass fit for making troches.

TINCTURES.

Tinctures should be digested in stopped glass bottles, and in a temperature of about 80°, unless otherwise directed. They should be frequently shaken during the preparation.

TINCTURE OF ALOES.

Take of Socotrine aloes in powder, half an ounce.
    Extract of liquorice, one ounce and a half.
    Alcohol, four fluidounces.
    Water, one pint.

Digest for ten days, and pour off the depurated tincture.

TINCTURE OF ALOES AND MYRRH.
FORMERLY " ELIXIR PROPRIETATIS."

Take of Myrrh in powder, two ounces.
    Alcohol, one pint and a half.
    Water, half a pint.

Misce alcohol cum aqua ; tum adde myrrham, digere per dies quinque, et demum adde

> Aloes socotrinæ in pulverem tritæ unciam unam cum semisse.
> Croci unciam unam.

Digere rursus per dies quinque, et tincturam defæcatum effunde.

———

TINCTURA AMMONIATA AROMATICA.

℞. Alcoholis ammoniati octantem dimidium.
Olei rorismarini fluidrachmam unam cum semisse.
Olei sassafras fluidrachmam unam.

Misce ut solvantur olea.

———

TINCTURA ANGUSTURÆ.

℞. Angusturæ contusæ uncias duas.
Alcoholis diluti, octantes duos.

Digere per dies decem, et per chartam cola.

———

TINCTURA ASSAFŒTIDÆ.

℞. Assafœtidæ uncias quatuor.
Alcoholis octantes duos.

Digere per dies decem, et cola.

———

TINCTURA CAMPHORÆ.

℞. Alcoholis diluti octantem unum.
Camphoræ unciam unam.

Misce ad camphoram solvendam.

Mix the alcohol with the water, then add the myrrh ; digest for five days ; and lastly, add of

Socotrine aloes in powder, an ounce and a half.
Saffron, one ounce.

Digest again for five days, and pour off the tincture from the sediment.

AMMONIATED AROMATIC TINCTURE.

Take of Ammoniated alcohol, half a pint.
Oil of rosemary, one fluidrachm and a half.
Oil of sassafras, one fluidrachm.

Mix them that the oils may be dissolved.

TINCTURE OF ANGUSTURA.

Take of Angustura in coarse powder, two ounces.
Diluted alcohol, two pints.

Digest for ten days, and filter.

TINCTURE OF ASSAFŒTIDA.

Take of Assafœtida, four ounces.
Alcohol, two pints.

Digest for ten days, and strain.

TINCTURE OF CAMPHOR.

Take of Alcohol, one pint.
Camphor, one ounce.

Mix, that the camphor may be dissolved.

TINCTURA CAMPHORÆ OPIATA.

℞. Opii ;
    Acidi benzoici ;
    Olei anisi ; utriusque drachmam unam.
    Glvcyrrhizæ extracti, unciam dimidiam.
    Mellis despumati uncias duas.
    Camphoræ scrupulos duos.
    Alcoholis diluti octantes duos.

Digere per dies decem, et cola.

TINCTURA CANTHARIDUM.

℞. Cantharidum contusarum drachmas tres.
    Alcoholis diluti octantes duos.

Digere per dies decem, et per chartam cola.

TINCTURA CAPSICI.

℞. Capsici unciam unam.
    Alcoholis diluti octantes duos.

Digere per dies decem, et per chartam cola.

TINCTURA CAPSICI ET CANTHARIDUM.

℞. Cantharidum contusarum drachmas decem.
    Capsici drachmam unam.
    Alcoholis diluti octantem unum.

Digere per dies decem, et per chartam cola.

OPIATED TINCTURE OF CAMPHOR.

FORMERLY PAREGORIC ELIXIR.

Take of Opium ;
      Benzoic acid ;
      Oil of anise, each one drachm.
      Liquorice, half an ounce.
      Clarified honey, two ounces.
      Camphor, two scruples.
      Diluted alcohol, two pints.

Digest for ten days, and filter.

TINCTURE OF CANTHARIDES.

Take of Cantharides bruised, three drachms.
      Diluted alcohol, two pints.

Digest for ten days, and strain.

TINCTURE OF CAYENNE PEPPER.

Take of Cayenne pepper, one ounce.
      Diluted alcohol, two pints.

Digest for ten days, and filter.

TINCTURE OF CAYENNE PEPPER AND CANTHA RIDES.

Take of Cantharides bruised, ten drachms.
      Cayenne pepper, one drachm.
      Diluted alcohol, one pint.

Digest for ten days, and filter.

TINCTURA CARDAMOMI.

℞. Cardamomi contusi uncias quatuor.
Alcoholis diluti octantes duos cum semisse.

Digere per dies decem, et per chartam cola.

TINCTURA CASTOREI.

℞. Castorei in pulverem triti uncias duas.
Alcoholis octantes duos.

Digere per dies decem, et per chartam cola.

TINCTURA CATECHU.

℞. Catechu uncias tres.
Cinnamomi contusi uncias duas.
Alcoholis diluti octantes duos.

Digere per dies decem, et per chartam cola.

TINCTURA CINCHONÆ.

℞. Cinchonæ in pulverem tritæ uncias sex.
Alcoholis diluti octantes duos cum semisse.

Digere per dies decem, et per chartam cola.

TINCTURE OF CARDAMOM.

Take of Cardamom bruised, four ounces.
Diluted alcohol, two pints and a half.

Digest for ten days, and filter.

TINCTURE OF CASTOR.

Take of Castor powdered, two ounces.
Alcohol, two pints.

Digest for ten days, and filter.

TINCTURE OF CATECHU.

Take of Catechu, three ounces.
Cinnamon bruised, two ounces.
Diluted alcohol, two pints.

Digest for ten days, and filter.

TINCTURE OF PERUVIAN BARK.

Take of Peruvian bark in coarse powder, six ounces.
Diluted alcohol, two pints and a half.

Digest for ten days, and filter.

29

TINCTURA CINCHONÆ COMPOSITA.

℞. Cinchonæ in pulverem tritæ uncias duas.
  Aurantii corticis exsiccati unciam unam cum semisse.
  Serpentariæ contusæ drachmas tres.
  Croci ;
  Santalini ; utriusque drachmam unam.
  Alcoholis diluti octantem unum cum semisse.

Digere per dies decem, et per chartam cola.

TINCTURA CINNAMOMI.

℞. Cinnamomi contusi uncias tres.
  Alcoholis diluti octantes duos cum semisse.

Digere per dies decem, et per chartam cola.

TINCTURA COLOMBÆ.

℞. Colombæ concisæ uncias duas cum semisse.
  Alcoholis diluti octantes duos.

Digere per dies decem, et per chartam cola.

TINCTURA DIGITALIS.

℞. Digitalis siccatæ uncias duas.
  Alcoholis diluti octantem unum.

Digere per dies decem, et per chartam cola.

COMPOUND TINCTURE OF PERUVIAN BARK.

Take of Peruvian bark powdered, two ounces.
       Orange peel dried, one ounce and a half.
       Virginia snakeroot bruised, three drachms.
       Saffron ;
       Red sanders, each one drachm.
       Diluted alcohol, one pint and a half.

Digest for ten days, and filter.

TINCTURE OF CINNAMON.

Take of Cinnamon bruised, three ounces.
       Diluted alcohol, two pints and a half.

Digest for ten days, and filter.

TINCTURE OF COLUMBO.

Take of Columbo sliced, two ounces and a half.
       Diluted alcohol, two pints.

Digest for ten days, and filter.

TINCTURE OF FOXGLOVE.

Take of Foxglove dried, two ounces.
       Diluted alcohol, one pint.

Digest for ten days, and filter.

TINCTURA ACETATIS FERRI.

℞. Potassæ acetatis ;
    Ferri sulphatis, utriusque unciam unam.
    Alcoholis octantem unum.

Contere potassæ acetatem et ferri sulphatem, mortario fictili, donec in massam coëant; hanc calore mediocri exsicca, et siccatam cum alcohole contere. Misturam in vase vitreo, bene obturato, per horas viginti quatuor digere, subinde agitans. Denique, quum fæces subsederint, liquorem limpidum effunde.

TINCTURA MURIATIS FERRI.

℞. Ferri carbonatis præcipitati libram dimidiam.
    Acidi muriatici libras tres.
    Alcoholis octantes tres.

Infunde ferri carbonati, in vase vitreo, acidum muriaticum ; misturam subinde per triduum agita ; deinde sepone, ut fæces, si quæ, subsideant, et liquorem effunde. Ad octantem unum ente vaporet hic : et frigefacto addetur alcohol.

TINCTURA GENTIANÆ.

℞. Gentianæ concisæ uncias duas.
    Aurantii corticis exsiccati unciam unam.
    Cardamomi contusi unciam dimidiam.
    Alcoholis diluti octantes duos.

Digere per dies decem, et per chartam cola.

TINCTURE OF ACETATE OF IRON.

Take of Acetate of potass ;
        Sulphate of iron, each one ounce.
        Alcohol, one pint.

Rub the acetate of potass and sulphate of iron in an earthen mortar until they unite into a soft mass, dry this with a moderate heat, and triturate it when dried, with the alcohol. Digest the mixture in a well-corked phial for twenty-four hours, shaking it occasionally. Lastly, after the fæces have subsided, pour off the limpid liquor.

TINCTURE OF MURIATE OF IRON.

Take of Precipitated carbonate of iron, half a pound.
        Muriatic acid, three pounds.
        Alcohol, three pints.

Pour the muriatic acid on the carbonate of iron in a glass vessel ; and shake the mixture occasionally during three days. Then set it by, that the fæces, if any, may subside, and pour off the liquor ; evaporate this slowly, to one pint, and when cold, add the alcohol.

TINCTURE OF GENTIAN.

Take of Gentian sliced, two ounces.
        Orange peel dried, one ounce.
        Cardamom bruised, half an ounce.
        Diluted alcohol, two pints.

Digest for ten days, and filter.

TINCTURA GUAIACI.

R. Guaiaci resinæ in pulverem tritæ libram unam.
Alcoholis octantes duos cum semisse.

Digere per dies decem, et per chartam cola.

TINCTURA GUAIACI AMMONIATA.

R. Guaiaci resinæ in pulverem tritæ uncias quatuor.
Alcoholis ammoniati octantem unum cum semisse.

Digere per dies decem, et per chartam cola.

TINCTURA HELLEBORI NIGRI.

R. Hellebori nigri concisi uncias quatuor.
Alcoholis diluti octantes duos.

Digere per dies decem, et per chartam cola.

TINCTURA HUMULI.

R. Humuli uncias quatuor.
Alcoholis octantem unum.

Ex humulo pulverem luteolum omnem **excute**, quem digere
per dies decem, et postea per chartam cola.

TINCTURE OF GUAIACUM.

Take of Resin of guaiacum in powder, one pound.
Alcohol, two pints and a half.

Digest for ten days, and filter.

AMMONIATED TINCTURE OF GUAIACUM.

Take of Resin of guaiacum in powder, four ounces.
Ammoniated alcohol, one pint and a half.

Digest for ten days, and filter.

TINCTURE OF BLACK HELLEBORE.

Take of Black hellebore sliced, four ounces.
Diluted alcohol, two pints.

Digest for ten days, and filter.

TINCTURE OF HOP.

Take of Hops, four ounces.
Alcohol one pint.

Beat out the yellow powder from the hops, and digest it ten days in the alcohol ; then filter.

TINCTURA HYOSCIAMI.

℞. Hyosciami siccati et in pulverem contusi uncias duas
cum quadrante.
Alcoholis diluti octantem unum.

Digere per dies decem, et per chartam cola.

TINCTURA JALAPÆ.

℞. Jalapæ in pulverem tritæ uncias octo.
Alcoholis diluti octantes duos.

Digere per dies decem, et per chartam cola.

TINCTURA KINO.

℞. Kino in pulverem tritæ uncias tres.
Alcoholis diluti octantes duos.

Digere per dies decem, et per chartam cola.

TINCTURA LAVANDULÆ.

℞. Spiritûs lavandulæ octantes tres.
Spiritûs rorismarini octantem unum.
Cinnamomi contusi unciam unam.
Caryophylli contusi drachmas duas.
Myristicæ contusæ unciam dimidiam.
Santalini rasi drachmas tres.

Digere per dies decem, et per chartam cola.

TINCTURE OF HENBANE.

Take of Henbane dried, and coarsely powdered, two ounces
and a quarter.
Diluted alcohol, one pint.

Digest for ten days, and filter.

TINCTURE OF JALAP.

Take of Jalap powdered, eight ounces.
Diluted alcohol, two pints.

Digest for ten days, and filter.

TINCTURE OF KINO.

Take of Kino powdered, three ounces.
Diluted alcohol, two pints.

Digest for ten days, and filter.

TINCTURE OF LAVENDER.

Take of Spirit of lavender, three pints.
Spirit of rosemary, one pint.
Cinnamon bruised, one ounce.
Cloves bruised, two drachms.
Nutmeg bruised, half an ounce.
Red sanders in shavings, three drachms.

Digest for ten days, and filter.

30

TINCTURA LOBELIÆ.

℞. Lobeliæ uncias duas.
Alcohoiis diluti octantem unum.

Digere per dies decem, et per chartam cola.

——◆——

TINCTURA MENTHÆ PIPERITÆ.

℞. Olei menthæ piperitæ fluidrachmas duas.
Alcoholis octantem unum.

Digere donec oleum cum alcohole rite permistum sit.

——◆——

TINCTURA MENTHÆ VIRIDIS.

℞ Olei menthæ viridis fluidrachmas duas.
Alcoholis octantem unum.

Digere donec oleum cum alcohole rite permistum sit.

——◆——

TINCTURA MOSCHI.

℞. Moschi drachmas duas.
Alcoholis octantem unum.

Digere per dies decem, et per chartam cola.

——◆——

TINCTURA MYRRHÆ.

℞. Myrrhæ in pulverem tritæ uncias tres.
Alcoholis fluiduncias viginti.
Aquæ fluiduncias decem.

Digere per dies decem, et per chartam cola.

TINCTURE OF INDIAN TOBACCO.

Take of Indian tobacco, two ounces.
  Diluted alcohol, one pint.

Digest for ten days, and filter.

TINCTURE OF PEPPERMINT.

Take of Oil of peppermint, two fluidrachms.
  Alcohol, one pint.

Digest till the oil is thoroughly blended with the alcohol.

TINCTURE OF SPEARMINT.

Take of Oil of spearmint, two fluidrachms.
  Alcohol, one pint.

Digest till the oil is thoroughly blended with the alcohol.

TINCTURE OF MUSK.

Take of Musk, two drachms.
  Alcohol, one pint.

Digest for ten days, and filter.

TINCTURE OF MYRRH.

Take of Myrrh in powder, three ounces.
  Alcohol, twenty fluidounces.
  Water, ten fluidounces.

Digest for ten days, and filter.

TINCTURA OPII.

℞. Opii in pulverem triti uncias duas.
Alcoholic diluti octantes duos.

Digere per dies decem, et per chartam cola

TINCTURA QUASSIÆ.

℞. Quassiæ rasæ unciam unam.
Alcoholis diluti octantes duos.

Digere per dies decem, et per chartam cola.

TINCTURA RHEI.

℞. Rhei contusi uncias tres.
Cardamomi contusi unciam dimidiam.
Alcoholis diluti octantes duos cum semisse.

Digere per dies decem, et per chartam cola.

TINCTURA RHEI ET ALOES.

℞. Rhei contusi drachmas decem.
Aloes socotrinæ tritæ drachmas sex.
Cardamomi contusi unciam dimidiam.
Alcoholis diluti octantes duos cum semisse.

Digere per dies decem, et per chartam cola.

TINCTURE OF OPIUM.

CALLED LAUDANUM.

Take of Opium powdered, two ounces.
Diluted alcohol, two pints.

Digest for ten days, and filter.

———•———

TINCTURE OF QUASSIA.

Take of Quassia rasped, one ounce.
Diluted alcohol, two pints.

Digest for ten days, and filter.

———•———

TINCTURE OF RHUBARB.

Take of Rhubarb bruised, three ounces.
Cardamom bruised, half an ounce.
Diluted alcohol, two pints and a half.

Digest for ten days, and filter.

———•———

TINCTURE OF RHUBARB AND ALOES.

FORMERLY "ELIXIR SACRUM."

Take of Rhubarb bruised, ten drachms.
Socotrine aloes in powder, six drachms.
Cardamom bruised, half an ounce.
Diluted alcohol, two pints and a half.

Digest for ten days, and filter.

TINCTURA RHEI ET GENTIANÆ.

℞. Rhei contusi uncias duas.
  Gentianæ concisæ et contusæ unciam dimidiam.
  Alcoholis diluti octantes duos cum semisse.

Digere per dies decem, et per chartam cola.

TINCTURA RHEI DULCIS.

℞. Rhei contusi uncias duas.
  Glycyrrhizæ contusæ ;
  Anisi contusi, utriusque unciam unam.
  Sacchari uncias duas.
  Alcoholis diluti octantes duos cum semisse.

Digere per dies decem, et per chartam cola.

TINCTURA SANGUINARIÆ.

℞. Sanguinariæ contusæ uncias duas.
  Alcoholis diluti octantem unum.

Digere per dies decem, et per chartam cola.

TINCTURA SAPONIS ET OPII.

℞. Saponis concisi uncias quatuor.
  Camphoræ uncias duas.
  Opii in pulverem triti unciam unam.
  Olei rorismarini unciam dimidiam.
  Alcoholis octantes duos.

Digere saponem et opium in alcohole per dies tres, tum cola, et colato camphoram et oleum adjice, et solve.

TINCTURE OF RHUBARB AND GENTIAN.

Take of Rhubarb in coarse powder, two ounces.
 Gentian sliced and bruised, half an ounce.
 Diluted alcohol, two pints and a half.

Digest for ten days, and filter.

SWEET TINCTURE OF RHUBARB.

Take of Rhubarb bruised, two ounces.
 Liquorice bruised ;
 Anise bruised, each one ounce.
 Sugar, two ounces.
 Diluted alcohol, two pints and a half.

Digest for ten days, and filter.

TINCTURE OF BLOODROOT.

Take of Bloodroot coarsely powdered, two ounces.
 Diluted alcohol, one pint.

Digest for ten days, and filter.

TINCTURE OF SOAP AND OPIUM.

Take of Soap in shavings, four ounces.
 Camphor, two ounces.
 Opium in powder, one ounce.
 Oil of rosemary, half an ounce.
 Alcohol, two pints.

Digest the soap and opium in the alcohol three days, then filter and add the camphor and oil, and dissolve.

TINCTURA SENNÆ AROMATICA.

℞. Sennæ drachmas duas.
　Coriandri ;
　Fœniculi singulorum drachmam unam.
　Santali drachmas duas.
　Croci ;
　Glycyrrhizæ utriusque drachmam dimidiam.
　Uvarum demptis acinis libram dimidiam.

Digere in octantibus duobus Alcoholis diluti per dies decem ;
dein cola, et octantem alterum alcoholis diluti iisdem adde ; per
dies quinque digere ; cola, et liquores misce.

TINCTURA SENNÆ COMPOSITA.

℞. Sennæ uncias tres.
　Jalapæ contusæ unciam unam.
　Coriandri ;
　Cari utriusque contusi unciam dimidiam.
　Cardamomi contusi drachmas duas.
　Alcoholis diluti octantes tres cum semisse.

Digere per dies decem, et colato adjice

　Sacchari uncias quatuor.

AROMATIC TINCTURE OF SENNA.

WARNER'S GOUT CORDIAL.

Take of Senna, two drachms.
    Coriander ;
    Fennel, each one drachm.
    Red sanders, two drachms.
    Saffron ;
    Liquorice, each half a drachm.
    Raisins stoned, half a pound.

Digest in two pints of diluted alcohol for ten days ; then strain, and add one other pint of diluted alcohol to the same ingredients ; digest for five days ; strain, and mix the liquor of both digestions.

COMPOUND TINCTURE OF SENNA.

FORMERLY " ELIXIR SALUTIS."

Take of Senna, three ounces.
    Jalap bruised, one ounce.
    Coriander ;
    Caraway, each bruised, half an ounce.
    Cardamom bruised, two drachms.
    Diluted alcohol, three pints and a half.

Digest for ten days, then filter, and add of

    Sugar, four ounces.

31

TINCTURA SERPENTARIÆ.

℞. Serpentariæ contusæ uncias duas.
Santali drachmam unam.
Alcoholis diluti octantes duos.

Digere per dies decem, et per chartam çola.

TINCTURA STRAMONII.

℞. Stramonii seminum contusorum uncias duas.
Alcoholis diluti octantem unum.

Digere per dies decem, et per chartam cola.

TINCTURA ACIDI SULPHURICI.

℞. Acidi sulphurici fluiduncias tres.
Alcoholis octantes duos.

Instilla acidum alcoholi paulatim. Misturam digere calore lenissimo, in vase clauso, per triduum ; dein adde

Zingiberis contusi unciam unam.
Cinnamomi contusi unciam unam cum semisse.

Digere rursus in vase clauso per septem dies ; dein per chartam, infundibulo vitreo impositam, cola.

TINCTURE OF VIRGINIA SNAKEROOT.

Take of Virginia snakeroot bruised, two ounces.
      Red sanders, one drachm.
      Diluted alcohol, two pints.

Digest for ten days, and filter.

TINCTURE OF THORNAPPLE.

Take of Thorn apple seeds bruised, two ounces.
      Diluted alcohol, one pint.

Digest for ten days, and filter.

TINCTURE OF SULPHURIC ACID.

FORMERLY ELIXIR OF VITRIOL.

Take of Sulphuric acid, three fluidounces.
      Alcohol, two pints.

Drop the acid gradually into the alcohol. Digest the mixture with a very gentle heat in a close vessel for three days, and then add of

      Ginger bruised, one ounce.
      Cinnamon bruised, one ounce and a half.

Digest again in a close vessel for seven days, and filter through paper placed in a glass funnel.

TINCTURA TOLUTANI.

℞. Tolutani unciam unam cum semisse.
Alcoholis octantem unum.

Digere donec solvatur tolutanum, et per chartam cola.

TINCTURA VALERIANÆ.

℞. Valerianæ uncias quatuor.
Alcoholis diluti octantes duos.

Digere per dies decem, et per chartam cola.

TINCTURA VALERIANÆ AMMONIATA.

℞. Valerianæ uncias quatuor.
Alcoholis ammoniati octantes duos.

Digere per dies decem, et per chartam cola.

TINCTURA VERATRI VIRIDIS.

℞. Veratri viridis contusi uncias octo.
Alcoholis diluti octantes duos cum semisse.

Digere per dies decem, et per chartam cola.

TINCTURE OF TOLU.

Take of Tolu, one ounce and a half.
Alcohol, one pint.

Digest till the tolu is dissolved, then filter.

TINCTURE OF VALERIAN.

Take of Valerian, four ounces.
Diluted alcohol, two pints.

Digest for ten days, and filter.

AMMONIATED TINCTURE OF VALERIAN.

Take of Valerian, four ounces.
Ammoniated alcohol, two pints.

Digest for ten days, and filter.

TINCTURE OF GREEN HELLEBORE.

Take of Green hellebore bruised, eight ounces.
Diluted alcohol, two pints and a half.

Digest for ten days, and filter.

UNGUENTA.

Unguenta parantur ex adipe vel oleo cum sevo vel cera, vel spermate ceti admixto. Crassitudinem butyri habere oportet, ut pulveres et medicamenta ponderosiora commixta non subsideant. Quoniam cuti illinenda sunt, mollia vel fluida in temperie corporis humani esse debent. Formulæ sequentes calori sexagesimum gradum non superanti adaptantur. Locis calidioribus cum ceræ vel sevi quantitate majore unguenta conficienda sint.

UNGUENTUM ACIDI NITROSI.

℞. Adipis libram unam.
   Acidi nitrosi fluidrachmas sex.

Acidum paulatim misce cum adipe liquefacto, et mixturam frigescentem diligenter subige.

UNGUENTUM AQUÆ ROSÆ.

℞. Amygdalæ olei fluiduncias duas.
   Spermatis ceti unciam dimidiam.
   Ceræ albæ drachmam unam.

Liquefac simul balneo aquoso, assidue movens, dein liquefactis adjice

   Aquæ rosæ fluiduncias duas ;

Et assidue move donec refrixerint.

OINTMENTS.

Ointments are prepared from lard or oil rendered of the consistence of butter by the addition of suet, wax, or spermaceti, so as to suspend the dry powders and more ponderous articles, with which they are frequently incorporated As they are to be applied to the skin, they should be soft or fluid at the temperature of the body. The following formulæ are calculated for a temperature not exceeding 60° Fahr. In a higher temperature more suet or wax may be added.

OINTMENT OF NITROUS ACID.

Take of Lard, one pound.
        Nitrous acid, six fluidrachms.

Mix the acid gradually with the melted lard, and diligently beat the mixture as it cools.

OINTMENT OF ROSEWATER.

Take of Oil of almonds, two fluidounces.
        Spermaceti, half an ounce.
        White wax, one drachm.

Melt the whole in a water bath, stirring it frequently ; when melted, add of

        Rose water, two fluidounces ;

And stir the mixture continually till it is cold.

UNGUENTUM CANTHARIDUM.

℞. Cantharidum in pulverem tritarum uncias duas.
Aquæ distillatæ fluiduncias octo.
Cerati resinosi uncias octo.

Aquam cum cantharidibus decoque ad dimidiam et cola ; liquori colato commisce ceratum, dein vaporet ad idoneam crassitudinem.

UNGUENTUM CUPRI SUBACETATIS.

℞. Unguenti simplicis partes quindecim.
Cupri subacetatis præparati in pulverem triti partem unam.

Unguento liquefacto adjice cuprum, et assidue move donec refrixerint.

UNGUENTUM GALLARUM.

℞. Gallarum in pulverem tritarum drachmam unam.
Adipis drachmas septem.

Adipi igne lento emollito pulverem adjice, et misce.

UNGUENTUM HYDRARGYRI.

℞. Hydrargyri purificati ;
Adipis, utriusque pondere partes tres.
Sevi partem unam.

Tere hydrargyrum diligenter in mortario cum pauxillo adipis donec evanescant globuli* dein adde reliquum adipis et sevi, bene interim omnia conterens.

* Globuli citius evanescent si hydrargyrus cum pauxillo unguenti jam antea parati seu adipis rancidi, seu terebinthinæ teretur.

OINTMENT OF CANTHARIDES.

Take of Cantharides in powder, two ounces.
          Distilled water, eight fluidounces.
          Resin cerate, eight ounces.

Boil the water with the cantharides to half its quantity, and strain. Mix the cerate into the strained liquor, and evaporate to a proper consistence.

OINTMENT OF THE SUBACETATE OF COPPER.

Take of Simple ointment, fifteen parts.
          Prepared subacetate of copper in powder, one part.

Melt the ointment, then add the copper, and mix them together.

OINTMENT OF GALLS.

Take of Galls in powder, one drachm.
          Lard, seven drachms.

Mix the powdered galls with the lard previously melted.

MERCURIAL OINTMENT.

Take of Purified mercury ;
          Lard, each three parts by weight.
          Suet, one part.

Rub the quicksilver carefully in a mortar with a small portion of the lard,* until the globules disappear ; then add the remainder of the lard and the suet, rubbing them well together.

* Employing a small portion of old ointment, of rancid lard, or of turpentine, greatly expedites the process.

32

UNGUENTUM HYDRARGYRI NITRATIS FORTIUS.

℞. Hydrargyri purificati partem unam.
Acidi nitrici partes duas.
Olei olivæ partes novem.
Adipis partes tres.

Solve hydrargyrum in acido, dein liquorem cum adipe et oleo prius simul liquefactis et denuo frigescentibus strenue subige in mortario vitreo, ut fiat unguentum.

UNGUENTUM HYDRARGYRI NITRATIS MITIUS.

Paratur eodem modo ex adipe et oleo triplici.

UNGUENTUM HYDRARGYRI NITRICO-OXIDI.

℞. Hydrargyri nitrico-oxidi partem unam.
Adipis partes octo.

Adipi liquefacto adjice oxidum et move donec refrixerint.

UNGUENTUM HYDRARGYRI OXIDI CINEREI

℞. Hydrargyri oxidi cinerei partem unam.
Adipis partes tres.

Adipi liquefacto adjice oxidum et misce.

OINTMENT OF NITRATE OF MERCURY.

Take of Purified mercury, by weight one part.
   Nitric acid, two parts.
   Olive oil, nine parts.
   Lard, three parts.

Dissolve the mercury in the acid, then mix the liquor with the oil and lard previously melted together, and just beginning to grow stiff. Stir them briskly together in a glass mortar, so as to form an ointment.

MILDER OINTMENT OF NITRATE OF MERCURY.

This is prepared in the same way, with three times the quantity of lard and oil.

OINTMENT OF THE NITRIC OXIDE OF MERCURY.

Take of Nitric oxide of mercury, one part.
   Lard, eight parts.

To the melted lard add the oxide, and mix them together until cool.

OINTMENT OF GREY OXIDE OF MERCURY.

Take of Grey oxide of mercury, one part.
   Lard, three parts.

Mix the oxide with the lard, previously melted.

UNGUENTUM HYDRARGYRI SUBMURIATIS AM-
MONIATI.

℞. Hydrargyri submuriatis ammoniati drachmam unam.
Adipis unciam unam cum semisse.

Adipi lento igne liquefacto adjice submuriatem hydrargyri ammoniatum et misce.

UNGUENTUM PICIS LIQUIDÆ.

℞. Picis liquidæ partes quinque.
Ceræ flavæ partes duas.

Liquefac simul et per linteum exprime.

UNGUENTUM PLUMBI SUBCARBONATIS.

℞. Unguenti simplicis libram unam.
Plumbi subcarbonatis uncias duas.

Unguento lento igne emollito adjice plumbum et misce donec refrixerint.

UNGUENTUM SIMPLEX.

℞. Ceræ albæ partes duas.
Olivæ olei partes quinque.

Liquefac simul lento igne, et assidue move donec refrixerint.

OINTMENT OF AMMONIATED SUBMURIATE OF MERCURY.

Take of Ammoniated submuriate of mercury, one drachm.
Lard, one ounce and a half.

To the melted lard add the ammoniated submuriate of mercury, and mix.

TAR OINTMENT.

Take of Tar, five parts.
Yellow wax, two parts.

Mix them together, and strain through linen.

OINTMENT OF SUBCARBONATE OF LEAD.

Take of Simple ointment, one pound.
Subcarbonate of lead, two ounces.

To the ointment previously softened add the lead, and stir them until cool.

SIMPLE OINTMENT.

Take of White wax, two parts.
Olive oil, five parts.

Melt them together and keep stirring until cool.

UNGUENTUM STRAMONII.

R. Stramonii foliorum recentium concisorum libras quinque.
Adipis libras quatuordecim.

Coque lento igne donec folia friabilia fiant, tum per linteum adipem exprime, et singulis hujus libris ; adjice,

Ceræ flavæ uncias duas.

Cera liquefacta, sinito gradatim concrescere ut fæces subsì-deant, quas ab unguento remove.

UNGUENTUM SULPHURIS.

R. Adipis partes quatuor.
Sulphuris partem unam.

Adipi liquefacto adjice sulphurem et misce.

UNGUENTUM SULPHURIS COMPOSITUM.

R. Sulphuris unciam unam.
Submuriatis hydrargyri ammoniati.
Acidi benzoici, utriusque drachmam unam.
Limonis olei fluidrachmam unam.
Acidi sulphurici minima sexaginta.
Potassæ nitratis drachmas duas.
Adipis libram dimidiam.

Adipi liquefacto adjice cætera, et misce donec refrixerint.

OINTMENT OF THORN APPLE.

Take of Thornapple leaves, fresh gathered and sliced, five
pounds.
Lard, fourteen pounds.

Let them simmer together over a gentle fire till the leaves
become crisp and dry, then press out the lard through a linen
cloth, and add to every pound of the compound, of

Yellow wax, two ounces.

When the wax is melted, let the whole be allowed to cool
gradually, that the impurities may subside, which must be separated from the ointment.

SULPHUR OINTMENT.

Take of Hogs lard, four parts.
Sulphur, one part.

Mix the sulphur with the melted lard.

COMPOUND SULPHUR OINTMENT.

Take of Sulphur, one ounce.
Ammoniated submuriate of mercury ;
Benzoic acid, each one drachm.
Oil of lemons, one fluidrachm.
Sulphuric acid, sixty minims.
Nitrate of potass, two drachms.
Lard, half a pound.

Melt the lard, then add the other articles, continually stirring
until the whole is cold.

UNGUENTUM VERATRI VIRIDIS.

R. Veratri viridis in pulverem triti uncias duos.
    Adipis uncias octo.
    Limonis olei minima viginti.

Adipi liquefacto adjice pulverem et oleum, et misce, assidue
movens donec refrixerint.
Eodem modo paratur unguentum veratri albi.

UNGUENTUM ZINCI OXIDI IMPURI.

R. Adipis partes quinque.
    Zinci oxidi impuri præparati partem unam.

Adipi liquefacto adjice oxidum et assidue move donec refrixerint.

VINA MEDICATA.

VINUM ALOES.

R. Aloes socotrinæ in pulverem tritæ unciam unam.
    Cardamomi contusi ;
    Zingiberis contusi, utriusque drachmam unam.
    Vini octantes duos.

Macera per dies decem, subinde agitans, et cola.

OINTMENT OF AMERICAN HELLEBORE.

Take of American hellebore in powder, two ounces.
  Lard, eight ounces.
  Oil of lemons, twenty minims.

To the lard previously melted add the oil and powder, continually stirring until cool.

In the same manner the ointment may be prepared of the white hellebore.

OINTMENT OF IMPURE OXIDE OF ZINC.

Take of Lard, five parts.
  Prepared impure oxide of zinc, one part.

To the melted lard add the zinc, and mix them together until cool.

MEDICATED WINES.

WINE OF ALOES.

Take of Socotrine aloes, in powder, one ounce.
  Cardamom, bruised ;
  Ginger, each one drachm.
  Wine, two pints.

Macerate for ten days, stirring occasionally, and afterwards strain.

VINUM ANTIMONII TARTARIZATI.

℞. Antimonii tartarizati scrupulos duos.
    Aquæ distillatæ bullientis fluiduncias quatuor.
    Vini fluiduncias sex.

Antimonium tartarizatum in aquâ distillatâ bulliente liqua ;
tum vinum adjice.

VINUM COLCHICI.

℞. Colchici recentis partem unam.
    Vini partes duas.

Macera per dies decem, et cola.

VINUM FERRI.

℞. Ferri ductilis consecti uncias quatuor.
    Vini octantes quatuor.

Ferrum vini octantibus duobus sparsum, donec rubigine coo-
pertum fuerit, äeri expone ; dein reliquum vini adde. Macera
per dies decem, subinde agitans, et cola.

VINUM GENTIANÆ COMPOSITUM.

℞. Gentianæ unciam dimidiam.
    Cinchonæ unciam unam.
    Aurantii corticis drachmas duas.
    Canellæ drachmam unam.
    Alcoholis diluti fluiduncias quatuor.
    Vini octantes duos cum semisse.

Radici atque corticibus concisis et contusis affunde primum
alcohol dilutum, et post horas viginti quatuor adde vinum ; tum
macera per dies decem, et cola.

WINE OF TARTARIZED ANTIMONY.

Take of Tartarized antimony, two scruples.
     Boiling distilled water, four fluidounces.
     Wine, six fluidounces.

Dissolve the tartarized antimony in the boiling distilled water ; then add the wine.

WINE OF MEADOW SAFFRON.

Take of Fresh meadow saffron, one part.
     Wine, two parts.

Macerate for ten days, and strain.

WINE OF IRON.

Take of Iron Wire cut in pieces, four ounces.
     Wine, four pints.

Sprinkle the wire with two pints of the wine, and expose it to the air until it be covered with rust ; then add the rest of the wine ; macerate for ten days, with occasional agitation, and filter.

COMPOUND WINE OF GENTIAN.

Take of Gentian, half an ounce.
     Peruvian bark, one ounce.
     Orange peel, two drachms.
     Canella, one drachm.
     Diluted alcohol, four fluidounces.
     Wine, two pints and a half.

First pour the diluted alcohol on the root and barks, sliced and bruised, and, after twenty-four hours, add the wine ; then macerate for ten days, and strain.

VINUM IPECACUANHÆ.

R. Ipecacuanhæ contusæ uncias duas.
Vini octantes duos.

Macera per dies decem, et per chartam cola-

VINUM OPII.

R. Opii uncias duas.
Cinnamomi contusi ;
Caryophylli contusi, utriusque drachmam unam.
Vini octantem unum.

Macera per dies decem, et cola.

VINUM RHEI.

R. Rhei concisi uncias duas.
Canellæ contusæ drachmam unam.
Alcoholis diluti fluiduncias duas.
Vini octantem unum.

Macera per dies decem, et per chartam cola.

VINUM TABACI.

R. Tabaci unciam unam.
Vini octantem unum.

Macera per dies decem, et per chartam cola.

VINUM VERATRI ALBI.

R. Veratri albi uncias quatuor.
Vini octantem unum.

Macera per dies decem, et per chartam cola.

WINE OF IPECACUANHA.

Take of Ipecacuanha bruised, two ounces.
    Wine, two pints.

Macerate for ten days, and strain.

WINE OF OPIUM.
CALLED SYDENHAM'S LAUDANUM.

Take of Opium, two ounces.
    Cinnamon, bruised ;
    Cloves bruised, each one drachm.
    Wine, one pint.

Macerate for ten days, and strain.

WINE OF RHUBARB.

Take of Rhubarb sliced, two ounces.
    Canella bruised, one drachm.
    Diluted alcohol, two fluidounces.
    Wine, one pint.

Macerate for ten days, and filter through paper.

WINE OF TOBACCO.

Take of Tobacco, one ounce.
    Wine, one pint.

Macerate for ten days, and filter.

WINE OF WHITE HELLEBORE.

Take of White hellebore, four ounces.
    Wine, one pint.

Macerate for ten days, and filter.

ZINCUM.

ZINCI ACETAS.

℞. Zinci sulphatis drachmam unam, in aquæ distillatæ fluidunciis decem soluti.

Plumbi acetatis scrupulos quatuor, in aquæ distillatæ fluidunciis decem soluti.

Misce liquores ut plumbi sulphas præcipitetur. Transfunde liquidum limpidum supernatans et vaporando crystallos elice.

ZINCI CARBONAS IMPURUS PRÆPARATUS.

℞. Zinci carbonatis impuri quantumvis.

Ure ; tum contere. Deinde fiat pulvis subtilissimus eodem modo, quo calcis carbonatem præparari præcipimus.

ZINCI OXIDUM.

Crucibulum amplum in furno prunis instructo ita collocetur ut hujus ostium versus paulo inclinet, et, cum illius fundus mediocriter canduerit, injiciatur zinci frustulum cuju pondus sit circiter unius drachmæ. Zincum brevi accendetur, et simul in floccos albos convertetur, qui subinde a metalli superficie spathulâ ferreâ retrahendi sunt, ut combustio ejus perfectius absolvatur ; et tandem, cessante flammâ, oxidum zinci e crucibulo auferendum est. Alio zinci frustulo tunc projecto, operatio iteretur, et, quoties opus fuerit, repetatur. Deinde oxidum zinci præparetur ut carbonas calcis.

ZINC.

ACETATE OF ZINC.

Take of Sulphate of zinc, one drachm, dissolved in ten fluidounces of distilled water.

Acetate of lead, four scruples, dissolved in ten fluidounces of distilled water.

Mix the solutions and a sulphate of lead will be precipitated. Decant the clear supernatant liquid, evaporate and crystallize.

PREPARED IMPURE CARBONATE OF ZINC.

CALLED PREPARED CALAMINE.

Take of Impure carbonate of zinc, any quantity.

Burn and break it small ; then let it be brought into the state
of a very fine powder, in the same manner that carbonate of
lime is prepared.

OXIDE OF ZINC.

FORMERLY FLOWERS OF ZINC.

Let a large crucible be placed in a furnace filled with live
coals, so as to be somewhat inclined towards its mouth ; and
when the bottom of the crucible is moderately red, throw into
it a small piece of zinc, about the weight of a drachm. The
zinc soon inflames, and is, at the same time, converted into
white flakes, which are to be from time to time removed from
the surface of the metal with an iron spatula, that the combustion may be more complete ; and at last, when the zinc ceases
to flame, the oxide of zinc is to be taken out of the crucible.
Having then put in another piece of zinc, the operation is to be
repeated, and may be repeated as often as is necessary. Lastly the oxide of zinc is to be prepared in the same way as the
carbonate of lime.

LATIN INDEX.

OF NAMES AND SYNONYMS.

34

ENGLISH INDEX.